Critical Care Assessment by M

Over the last ten years, pregnancy has not only become more complicated for many women, but the traditional provision of general intensive care units has been reduced. To bridge this gap, critical care units, usually staffed by midwives, have been set up in many maternity units. This textbook is an accessible and comprehensive introduction to this emerging area of practice.

Critical Care Assessment by Midwives also notably sets out a template for assessment of women that will enable early identification of deteriorating health. Serious illness can arise subsequent to an emergency, a pre-existing illness or a complication of pregnancy but can also occur in the context of what appears to be a low risk pregnancy. For this reason, all midwives need to be skilled in assessment that facilitates timely, appropriate referrals and saves lives.

It covers:

- ABCDE assessment tailored for midwives;
- assessment of cardiac conditions;
- assessment of respiratory conditions;
- assessment of neurological conditions;
- pre-eclampsia;
- haemorrhage;
- shock, including hypovolaemia, sepsis and anaphylaxis;
- haemodynamic monitoring;
- fluid replacement and balance;
- ketoacidosis, hypoglycaemia and sickle cell crisis.

Covering the context of care, relevant pathophysiology, signs and symptoms, specific assessment in detail, relevant drugs, assessment of the fetus, summaries of management, psychosocial support and the specific professional responsibilities of the midwife, this is an essential guide for all midwives and midwifery students.

Maureen Boyle is a Senior Lecturer in Midwifery at the University of West London, UK.

Judy Bothamley is a Senior Lecturer in Midwifery at the University of West London, UK.

Critical Care Assessment by Midwives

Maureen Boyle and
Judy Bothamley

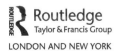
Routledge
Taylor & Francis Group

LONDON AND NEW YORK

First published 2018
by Routledge
2 Park Square, Milton Park, Abingdon, Oxon OX14 4RN

and by Routledge
711 Third Avenue, New York, NY 10017

Routledge is an imprint of the Taylor & Francis Group, an informa business

© 2018 Maureen Boyle and Judy Bothamley

The right of Maureen Boyle and Judy Bothamley to be identified as authors of this work has been asserted by them in accordance with sections 77 and 78 of the Copyright, Designs and Patents Act 1988.

British Library Cataloguing-in-Publication Data
A catalogue record for this book is available from the British Library

Library of Congress Cataloging-in-Publication Data
Names: Boyle, Maureen, author. | Bothamley, Judy, author.Title: Critical care assessment by midwives / Maureen Boyle and Judy Bothamley.
Description: New York, NY : Routledge, 2018. | Includes bibliographical references and index.
Identifiers: LCCN 2018009667| ISBN 9781138740204 (hbk) | ISBN 9781138740259 (pbk.) | ISBN 9781315183657 (ebk)
Subjects: | MESH: Pregnancy Complications | Critical Care | Needs Assessment | Midwifery
Classification: LCC RG571 | NLM WQ 240 | DDC 618.3—dc23
LC record available at https://lccn.loc.gov/2018009667

ISBN: 978-1-138-74020-4 (hbk)
ISBN: 978-1-138-74025-9 (pbk)
ISBN: 978-1-315-18365-7 (ebk)

Typeset in Sabon and GillSans
by Florence Production Ltd, Stoodleigh, Devon, UK

Disclaimer
This book contains information obtained from authentic and highly-regarded sources. While all reasonable efforts have been made to publish reliable data and information, neither the authors nor the publisher can accept any legal responsibility or liability for any errors or omissions that may be made. The publishers wish to make clear that any views or opinions expressed in this book by individual authors are personal to them and do not necessarily reflect the views/opinions of the publishers. The information or guidance contained in this book is intended for use by medical, scientific or healthcare professionals and is provided strictly as a supplement to the medical or other professional's own judgement, their knowledge of the patient's medical history, relevant manufacturer's instructions and the appropriate best practice guidelines. Because of the rapid advances in medical science, any information or advice on dosages, procedures or diagnoses should be independently verified. The reader is strongly urged to consult the relevant national drug formulary and the drug companies' and device or material manufacturers' printed instructions, and their websites, before administering or utilising any of the drugs, devices or materials mentioned in this book. This book does not indicate whether a particular treatment is appropriate or suitable for a particular individual. Ultimately, it is the sole responsibility of the medical professional to make his or her own professional judgements, so as to advise and treat patients appropriately. The authors and publishers have also attempted to trace the copyright holders of all material reported in this publication and apologise to copyright holders if permission to publish in this form has not been obtained. If any copyright material has not been acknowledged please write and let us know that so we may rectify in any future reprint.

Contents

Illustrations

Figures

Tables

Boxes

Abbreviations

ABG	arterial blood gases
ACS	acute chest syndrome
AFE	amniotic fluid embolism
AFLP	acute fatty liver of pregnancy
CNS	central nervous system
CRP	C-reactive protein
CS	Caesarean section
CSF	cerebral spinal fluid
CT	computed tomography
CTG	cardiotocography
CVA	cerebrovascular accident
DIC	disseminated intravascular coagulation
DOB	date of birth
DVT	deep vein thrombosis
ECF	extracellular fluid
ECG	electrocardiogram
ECHO	echocardiogram
FBC	full blood count (haemoglobin, white blood cells and platelets).
FFP	fresh frozen plasma
FHR	fetal heart rate
GA	general anaesthetic
GCS	Glasgow Coma Score
HDU	high dependency unit
HELLP	haemolysis, elevated liver enzymes, low platelets
ICF	intracellular fluid
ICP	intracranial pressure
ICU	intensive care unit
LMWH	low molecular weight heparin
LOC	loss of consciousness
MC&S	microscopy, culture & sensitivity
MDT	multidisciplinary team
MEOWS	modified early obstetric warning scoring systems
MI	myocardial infarction
MRI	magnetic resonance imaging

PCR   protein:creatinine ratio
PE   pulmonary embolism
PET   pre-eclampsia
RCOG   Royal College of Obstetricians and Gynaecologists
RFT   renal function tests
SAH   subarachnoid haemorrhage
SL   sublingual (usually concerning administration of drugs)
SLE   systemic lupus erythematosus
SOB   shortness of breath
TEDS   thromboembolic deterrent stockings
U&E   urea and electrolytes
UKOSS   UK Obstetric Surveillance System
USS   ultrasound scan

Introduction

Childbirth is normally an exciting physiological life event for women and their families. However, complications occur even in the context of what appears to be an uncomplicated birth. Midwives are now more likely to care for women with complex medical conditions due to improvements in medical care generally, women having children at an older age, increased prevalence of conditions such as diabetes and obesity and the increase in reproductive technologies. These women require the same standard of care for both their pregnancy and medical needs, and midwives who are confident in critical care assessment are well-placed to provide this holistic care.

Back-to-basics approach

Reports from the 'Confidential enquiry into maternal deaths' over recent years have been a reminder of the need for a 'back-to-basics' approach[1,2,3] that involves taking basic observations, recognising when they are abnormal and getting the right help. All health professionals working with pregnant and postpartum women are included in the recommendations of these reports, but midwives face some unique challenges to this approach. The assessment of routine observations is often delegated to maternity support workers, which prevents the midwife from benefitting from the subtleties of holistic assessment that comes from doing it themselves. The fast pace of clinical practice, the reduction in postnatal visits and the complexity of the social and medical features of the women being cared for all create an environment that can conspire against the opportunity to make a thorough and considered assessment. The focus on 'normality' by midwives has led to problems in the recognition of deteriorating ill health.[4] Midwives have expressed anxiety with regard to caring for women who are unwell, and may feel unprepared for that role.[5] The use of MEOWS charts with triggers for escalating care has attempted to address this. However, education, experience and common sense, as well as physically observing and talking to the woman, are all still needed to identify that something is 'not quite right'.

Chain of prevention

Smith[6] originally coined the phrase 'chain of prevention' in relation to averting in-hospital cardiac arrests. The features of this chain (Figure I.1) are relevant in maternity care settings, and sum up the main messages of this book. The woman's care is dependent on the strength of all links in the chain.

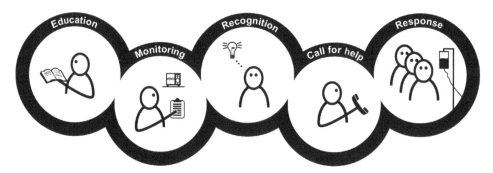

Figure 1.1 Chain of prevention

Source: Reproduced with the permission of professor GB Smith (from Smith, GB. 2010. In-Hospital Cardiac Arrest: Is It Time for an In-Hospital 'Chain of Prevention'? *Resuscitation, 81*(9): 1209–11)

Education of midwives in assessment, recording and interpreting vital signs, identifying signs of deteriorating ill-health and escalating appropriately is the crucial front-line start of the chain. Multidisciplinary learning – where doctors, midwives and nurses learn to understand and respect each other's roles, skills and perspectives – is advocated.[7] Midwives need to feel confident in their skills of assessment, and education will help fill any gaps in training.

The quality of appropriate *monitoring* frequency and recording of observations forms the second link. Chapter 1 specifies the details of ABCDE assessment, Chapter 2 explains haemodynamic monitoring and Chapter 3 examines fluid balance. Subsequent chapters – Chapter 7 (Assessment of the respiratory system), Chapter 8 (Assessment of the cardiac system) and Chapter 9 (Assessment of the neurological system) – provide system-specific assessment detail.

The early *recognition* of a woman at risk of critical illness relies on the detection of subtle changes in her physiology as the body starts to compensate. It is a window of opportunity to prevent serious morbidity and mortality. However, pregnant women have good physiological reserve and therefore compensate well until a point of abrupt deterioration.[7] The emphasis throughout the book is on assessment to identify a deteriorating condition, and Chapter 4 (Shock), Chapter 5 (Haemorrhage) and Chapter 6 (Pre-eclampsia) look specifically at the challenges of identifying these more common obstetric problems. MEOWS (modified early obstetric warning system/signs/scores) were introduced following the 'Saving mothers' lives' report of 2003–5.[1] Recommendations to use MEOWS charts are discussed throughout the book when referring to how vital signs and other observations should be recorded. This form of record-keeping has, however, been called by other names; for example, MEWS (modified early-warning signs/score/system) or MOEWS (modified obstetric early-warning signs/score/system). Whatever the name given to these 'trigger' and 'alert' charts, they all generally contain the same information and are helpful for the observation of trends, which is so important in identifying women whose condition is deteriorating.

Calling for help from appropriate senior staff at the earliest stage of deterioration will improve outcomes for women. Effective team working relationships, efficient systems of calling for assistance and good communication with medical staff based on objective assessment will aid the effectiveness of timely referral. A number of areas of improvements in *response* have occurred in recent years, including improvements noted since the introduction of multidisciplinary emergency simulation training and the use of critical outreach teams, which have been valuable in improving standards of care. The midwife's role in response will focus on initial life-saving actions, ongoing assessment, important psychological support for the women and carrying out treatment plans.

Critical care

The Department of Health report 'Comprehensive critical care'[8] recommended that the terms 'high dependency' and 'intensive care' be replaced with the term 'critical care'. This report proposed that the care required by an individual should be independent of location. The term 'critical care without walls' was coined.[9] This is particularly relevant for maternity care where there are two areas of specialty: the normal

---

Box 1.1 Summary of classifications of care[10] with examples pertinent to maternity care

Level of care	Basic description	Maternity example
Level 0	Normal care	Care of low-risk women
Level 1	Women at risk of their condition deteriorating and needing additional monitoring, or those recently relocated from higher levels of care	Risk of haemorrhage Oxytocin infusion Pre-eclampsia on oral anti-hypertensives or fluid restriction Women with medical conditions
Level 2	Single organ support Women requiring invasive monitoring/intervention that includes support for a single failing organ system (excluding advanced respiratory support)	Basic respiratory support including continuous positive airway pressure (CPAP) Cardiovascular support: IV anti-hypertensives, use of CVP and/or arterial lines, vasoactive medication Neurological support; magnesium infusion to control seizures Management of acute fulminant hepatic failure such as HELLP syndrome or acute fatty liver of pregnancy
Level 3	Women requiring advanced respiratory support (mechanical ventilation)	Invasive mechanical ventilation Support of two or more organ systems

requirements for childbirth with the involvement of midwives and obstetricians, alongside support of critical illness requiring specialist doctors and nurses in critical care. The obstetric anaesthetist is an important link and should be involved at early stages of escalation of concerns. Box I.1 indicates the levels of classification of care. Local facilities and staff expertise will determine where and by whom care will be provided when women develop specialist critical care requirements. The use of critical care outreach teams has been a welcome innovation, enabling expertise to come to the labour ward and facilitate the support for midwives, obstetricians and obstetric anaesthetists in escalation and decision-making and access to the best care for women.

References

1. Lewis, G (ed.). 2007. The confidential enquiry into maternal and child health (CEMACH). Saving mothers' lives: reviewing maternal deaths to make motherhood safer – 2003–2005. The seventh report on confidential enquiries into maternal deaths in the United Kingdom. London: CEMACH.
2. Centre for Maternal and Child Enquiries (CMACE). 2011. Saving mothers' lives: reviewing maternal deaths to make motherhood safer: 2006–2008. The eighth report on confidential enquiries into maternal deaths in the United Kingdom. *British Journal of Obstetrics and Gynaecology, 118*(1): 1–203.
3. Knight, M, Nair, M, Tuffnell, D, Kenyon, S, Shakespeare, J, Brocklehurst, P and Kurinczuk, JJ (eds) on behalf of MBRRACE-UK. 2016. *Saving lives, improving mothers' care: surveillance of maternal deaths in the UK 2012–2014 and lessons learned to inform maternity care from the UK and Ireland confidential enquiries into maternal deaths and morbidity 2009–2014*. Oxford, UK: National Perinatal Epidemiology Unit, University of Oxford.
4. Kirkup, B. 2015. The report of the Morecambe Bay investigation. Available at www.gov.uk/government/publications/morecambe-bay-investigation-report. Accessed 9 September 2017.
5. Eadie, IJ and Sheridan, NF. 2017. Midwives' experiences of working in an obstetric high dependency unit: a qualitative study. *Midwifery, 47*(April): 1–7.
6. Smith, GB. 2010. In-hospital cardiac arrest: is it time for an in-hospital 'chain of prevention'? *Resuscitation, 81*(9): 1209–11.
7. Gauntlett, R on behalf of the MBRRACE-UK critical chapter writing group. 2016. Messages for critical care. In: Knight, M, Nour, M, Tuffnell, D, Kenyon, S, Shakespeare, J, Brocklehurst, P and Kurinczuk, JJ (eds) on behalf of MBRRACE-UK. *Saving lives, improving mothers' care: surveillance of maternal deaths in the UK 2012–2014 and lessons learned to inform maternity care from the UK and Ireland confidential enquiries into maternal deaths and morbidity 2009–2014*. Oxford, UK: National Perinatal Epidemiology Unit, University of Oxford, pp. 83–95.
8. Department of Health. 2000. Comprehensive critical care: a review of adult critical care services. Available at http://webarchive.nationalarchives.gov.uk/+/http://www.dh.gov.uk/en/Publicationsandstatistics/Publications/PublicationsPolicyAndGuidance/DH_4006585. Accessed 24 September 2017.
9. Hillman, K. 2002. Critical care without walls. *Current Opinion in Critical Care, 8*(6): 594–9.
10. Royal College of Anaesthetists (RCOA). 2011. Providing equity of critical and maternity care for the critically ill pregnant or recently pregnant woman. Available at www.rcoa.ac.uk/system/files/CSQ-ProvEqMatCritCare.pdf.

Chapter 1

Structured assessment to identify deteriorating health

Introduction

A number of reports,[1,2,3] including the 'Confidential enquiry into maternal deaths',[4,5] have noted the need for earlier identification of women who are becoming unwell and for seamless care to support their recovery. While there has been considerable improvement in dealing with obstetric emergencies,[6] other complications can occur, even in the context of what appears to be an uncomplicated birth. There remains a need for midwives to recognise signs of deteriorating illness and refer appropriately.

It has been noted that it is more difficult to detect if a pregnant woman is becoming unwell. They are generally young and healthy with good physiological reserve, enabling them to compensate well. Some of the symptoms of ill health, such as breathlessness, may be normal for pregnancy. The progression of illness can be quicker, such as the extent of blood loss in postpartum haemorrhage. The expectation of normality in maternity settings may be a factor towards delays in initiating referral.[7] Midwives are not responsible for making the diagnosis but for performing the right observations at suitably frequent intervals, recording them accurately, giving some initial care and ensuring that the right medical staff respond to review the woman. These actions by the midwife will be life-saving.

Physiology

Understanding the signs of compensatory mechanisms indicative of deteriorating health is required to address health problems early and avert serious morbidity and mortality (see Chapter 4 for more details of the physiology of compensatory mechanisms). Table 1.1 summarises the physiological changes in pregnancy that need to be considered when assessing the critically ill woman who is pregnant or has recently given birth.

Table 1.1 Physiological changes to be considered when assessing the critically ill woman who is pregnant or has recently given birth[1,8,9]

	Changes in pregnancy	*Factors to consider with regard to assessment of critical ill health*
Cardiovascular system		
Plasma volume	Up to 50% plasma volume expansion	Physiological anaemia; reduced oxygen-carrying capacity; check haemoglobin levels.
Heart rate	Increased by 15–20 bpm	Check against baseline for individual woman; note trends.
Cardiac output and venous return	Increased by 40–50% by term Supine hypotension syndrome occurs when the gravid uterus impedes inferior vena cava and venous return	Women can tolerate quite large amounts of blood loss postnatally without change to blood pressure but this will vary; check vital signs to identify compensatory changes. Women should be cared for lying on their side or with left lateral tilt to optimise cardiac output.
Uterine blood flow	Significant increase during pregnancy of up to 10% of cardiac output	Potential for large volumes of blood loss quickly, particularly around the time of delivery of the placenta; concealed blood loss both antenatally and following surgery can occur; inaccuracies of estimated blood loss may lead to underestimation of the severity of blood loss.
Systemic vascular resistance	Decreased in pregnancy due to effects of progesterone, resulting in general vasodilation	The response of peripheral vasoconstriction and other features of compensatory mechanisms will mask features of shock until the woman is significantly unwell. Perform observations and plot on MEOWS chart.
Coagulation	Pregnancy is a pro-coagulant state	Concentration of clotting factors after delivery and reduced venous return increases risk of venous thromboembolism (VTE). Risk assessment for VTE and prophylaxis is required.
Tendency for anaemia	Haemodilution results in physiological anaemia Increased fetal requirements for iron	Women may have poor iron stores and this combined with physiological changes may leave women with iron deficiency anaemia. Haemorrhage may exacerbate this, reducing oxygen-carrying capacity. Check oxygen saturations and haemoglobin levels.

continued

Table 1.1 continued

	Changes in pregnancy	*Factors to consider with regard to assessment of critical ill health*
Respiratory system		
Airway changes Laryngeal oedema	Fluid shift and generalised vasodilation	Increased mucosal oedema Laryngeal oedema can make intubation more difficult. Airway assessment
Oxygen consumption	Increased by 20% due to metabolic demand of fetus and increased requirements of pregnancy	Increased oxygen requirements and changes in lung function make the pregnant woman become hypoxic more readily. Check oxygen saturations
Respiratory rate and ventilation	Increased respiratory rate Gravid uterus causes displacement of the diaphragm Changes in lung function – residual capacity reduced	Breathlessness is a common sign in a healthy pregnancy and this may mean that breathlessness as a sign of critical ill health is 'explained away' as normal (see Chapter 7 for assessment of breathlessness). Ventilation more difficult
Arterial pCO_2	Decreased buffering capacity, making acidosis more likely	Note any increase in respiratory rate.
Other changes		
Reduced gastric motility and relaxation of lower oesophageal sphincter	Due to effects of progesterone Increased risk of aspiration of stomach contents	Minor disorder symptoms of pregnancy, including heartburn and nausea, may be confused with more serious presentation of illness such as chest pain and liver disease. Intubation with effective cricoid pressure and the use of H_2 antagonists and antacids prophylactically is recommended.
Uterus	Increased blood supply, interventions in labour and area for healing left by placenta predispose to haemorrhage and infection	Need for close monitoring of uterine contraction and signs of bleeding and infection, particularly in the postnatal period.
Urinary system	Vasodilation effects of progesterone and pressure from enlarging uterus	Increased risk of urinary tract infection (UTI) Asymptomatic bacteriuria more common Frequent urinalysis
Fluid balance	Increased oncotic pressure; fluid shift changes, which creates increased risk of generalised oedema At risk of pulmonary oedema	Monitoring of fluid intake, urine output and assessment of fluid balance Fluid restriction may be required. Respiratory assessment

continued

Table 1.1 continued

	Changes in pregnancy	Factors to consider with regard to assessment of critical ill health
Fetus		Deterioration of fetal wellbeing is a sensitive indicator of maternal health.

Fetus may need to be delivered to improve outcome for a critically ill mother. |
| Breastfeeding | | Consideration regarding suitability of postnatal medication |
| Psychological impact | Expectations of childbirth as normal physiology event

Adaption to parenting | Psychological support and assessment |

Table 1.2 lists some of the more common acute illnesses that may occur in the maternity setting, with a summary of the presenting signs the midwife might note. What is notable in this list is the similarity of changes in basic observations as indicators of development of critical ill health. Subsequent chapters will elaborate on the features of particular illnesses.

Structured assessment by the midwife

The simple pneumonic ABC was originally used for assessment of collapse in the context of the need for cardiopulmonary resuscitation. An extended version is now advocated as a structured approach to identify early signs of deterioration.[10] Midwives will use a combination of ABCDE (see Box 1.1) and traditional midwifery head-to-toe assessment (largely summed up under E). Some priorities will vary, such as the midwife being more likely to look for bleeding and assess uterine contraction in a postnatal woman as a precedence to other assessments apart from airway and level of consciousness. Stemming bleeding from an atonic uterus by rubbing up a contraction is the most common emergency procedure carried out by midwives. A review of pain

---

Box 1.1 Summary of ABCDE[10]

A: assess *airway* and treat if required;

B: assess *breathing* and treat if required;

C: assess *circulation* and treat if required;

D: assess *disability* (level of consciousness) and respond as required;

E: *expose* and *examine* the woman using traditional midwifery head-to-toe assessment once ABCD are stable. This will include assessment of fetal wellbeing.

Table 1.2 Summary of examples of acute illness and presenting features

Example of acute illness	Pathophysiological changes	Signs that indicate deteriorating health
Hypovolaemic shock e.g. PPH, APH	Excessive blood loss reducing circulating blood volume	Raised RR, HR, peripheral vasoconstriction
Severe sepsis	Inflammatory reaction to infection causing vasodilation	Raised HR, RR Lowered BP Peripheral vasoconstriction Raised or lowered temperature
Myocardial infarction	Blockage of coronary artery leading to ischaemic damage to heart muscle interfering with the pump action of the heart	Raised HR, RR, BP and peripheral vasoconstriction Pain
Pulmonary embolism (PE)	Blood clot that has travelled from another part of the body that blocks blood flow to part of the lung, causing significant problems with blood oxygenation	*Minor PE* Pleuritic chest pain Breathlessness Raised HR May cough up blood *Major PE* Severe breathlessness Central chest pain Collapse Cardiac arrest
Acute asthma	Hypoxaemia Bronchoconstriction caused by narrowing of airways	Raised respiratory rate, HR and BP Use of accessory muscles
Pre-eclampsia	Endothelial damage leading to multi-organ dysfunction	Varied range of symptoms Raised BP (may be normal) Protein in urine Oedema Headache, visual disturbances, epigastric pain (often asymptomatic)
Amniotic fluid embolism	Anaphylaxis-like inflammatory response to amniotic fluid entering the maternal circulation, causing sudden collapse with impairment of coagulation	Shortness of breath Altered mental status Reduced BP Cardiovascular collapse Disseminated intravascular coagulation (DIC)
Diabetic ketoacidosis	Raised blood sugar due to lack of insulin Cell starvation	Raised RR (smell of acetone), HR Lowered BP Polyuria, glycosuria

Abbreviations: APH – antepartum haemorrhage; BP – blood pressure; HR – heart rate; PPH – postpartum haemorrhage; RR – respiratory rate is another important aspect of initial assessment. Chest pain accompanied by breathlessness, constant abdominal pain or tenderness that is not relieved by usual analgesia, severe headaches and unilateral leg pain are all examples of pain that should prompt the midwife to seek urgent medical review.

Midwifery assessment of a woman will therefore involve:

- a quick review of airway and breathing;
- a check for contraction of the uterus postnatally (tone of the uterus antenatally) and assessment for any signs of bleeding;
- a review of any significant pain (see Box 1.2);
- assessment of the woman's current condition by performing a physical examination that will include a set of basic observations in line with an ABCD-structured approach;
- a review of the woman's history and assessment of any risk factors;
- a traditional head-to-toe midwifery assessment (E), which will include assessment of the fetus or examination of the newborn once any life-threatening problems have been addressed.

The midwife should initiate a set of basic observations at any point that an assessment is indicated (see Box 1.3). This might be when a woman is admitted because

---

Box 1.2 Useful questions about pain

— Describe the pain. Is it sharp, dull, aching, hot, tight?

— Is it constant or intermittent?

— Where is it? Put a finger where the pain is worst. Does the pain go anywhere?

— Does anything bring on the pain?

— Does anything help the pain? Have you taken anything?

Box 1.3 Summary of key assessments

- Vital signs;
- Temperature, pulse, respiratory rate, responsiveness;
- Blood pressure;
- Oxygen saturation monitoring;
- Further assessments;
- Pain assessment (see Box 1.2);

- Urine output and urine tests;
- Breasts, uterus, lochia, vaginal loss, legs;
- Skin perfusion, capillary refill;
- Neurological function;
- Blood sugar level;
- Fetal wellbeing if antenatal.

she is unwell, following surgery or as part of ongoing assessment when known to be unwell. Midwives sometimes instigate assessment based on intuition that the woman is 'not quite right'. The woman herself or family members may prompt the midwife by expressing a feeling that things are not right. Intuition arises from experience, where patterns are observed from previous experiences, and the midwife should follow up with a more objective assessment. In many hospital situations, the taking of observations is delegated to maternity care assistants. When the midwife is concerned about the woman, it is essential that the midwife does this assessment. Subtle changes such as a bounding or thready pulse will be felt. When the pulse is taken, what does her skin feel like? Cold, hot, clammy, sweaty? Does she look pale or flushed? Is any rash evident? Can the midwife detect any unusual odours – offensive lochia, the smell of diarrhoea?

ABCDE assessment

A quick assessment of airway, breathing, circulation and level of consciousness (ABCD) is fundamental to midwifery assessment. However, in most cases of assessment for deteriorating health, the woman will be conscious and able to talk and the midwife will need to elicit more subtle features of deteriorating condition.

A: Airway

Many aspects of initial ABCD assessment can be ascertained by observing the woman and asking the question 'How are you?'

The evaluation of the woman's response to this question covers a number of aspects of initial assessment, both in the content of her response and the physical aspects of the way she communicates. To respond verbally, the woman must have a patent airway and circulating oxygenated blood. She must have reasonable respiratory effort to be able to produce a response and she must have adequate cerebral function to comprehend and answer. However, does she have to pause to breathe, or find it difficult to talk? This will indicate increased respiratory effort and give an indication of her level of pain. Does her response indicate any level of confusion or neurological impairment?

B: Breathing

A change in respiratory status is a sensitive indicator of deteriorating illness due to respiratory, metabolic, cardiovascular or neurological conditions (see Chapter 7 for detailed assessment of the respiratory system). The midwife should observe for signs of increased respiratory effort, such as use of accessory muscles, difficulty in completing sentences or pausing in-between words. Observe for abnormal sounds such as stridor, gurgling, wheezing and any abnormal sputum production. The importance of assessing and recording the respiratory rate cannot be overemphasised. A respiratory rate of over 20 breaths per minute is cause for concern, and a rate of over 30 breaths per minute is a sign of significant pathology, necessitating immediate action. Using a pulse oximetry, if available, is a quick and useful way to assess respiratory function, giving valuable information concerning oxygen saturation. Always record whether the woman is breathing room air or oxygen when the reading is taken; if the latter, record the flow of oxygen the woman is receiving at the time of the reading. If oxygen saturation is below 95%, oxygen therapy is indicated. Measurement of arterial blood gases may be required, as an increased respiratory rate can indicate developing acidosis (see Chapter 2 for more detail of haemodynamic monitoring).

C: Circulation

A functioning circulatory system will deliver essential oxygenated blood to the tissues. As haemorrhage is a common cause of hypovolaemic shock related to childbirth, the evaluation of blood loss and the tone of the uterus will be essential aspects of the circulation assessment. Steps to control the bleeding are fundamental to preserving the health of the woman. However, there are other causes of deficiencies in circulation, including concealed blood loss, cardiac disorders and sepsis. Attaining pulse rate, blood pressure and assessment of perfusion provide vital initial information. Nothing replaces making these assessments manually, although use of equipment will aid ongoing assessment. When assessing the vital signs, note the woman's *general appearance*. The woman who looks pale is displaying signs of sympathetic mediated vasoconstriction as the body diverts blood away from the peripheries to conserve blood pressure to vital organs. She may feel cold and clammy to the touch when her *pulse* is taken. A weak, thready pulse may indicate hypovolaemia, and a strong, bounding pulse can be associated with the vasodilation of early stages of sepsis or anaphylaxis. An irregular pulse should be followed up with a 12 lead ECG. Record her temperature. A raised or low temperature can indicate infection, with a low temperature associated with severe sepsis.

Assessment of *blood pressure* is included. Midwives will be familiar with identifying a raised blood pressure (above 140/90 mmHg) that may be associated with pre-eclampsia (PET). See Chapter 6 for detailed assessment of PET, whereby blood pressure is assessed within the context of a urine test for protein, symptoms of epigastric pain, severe headache and visual disturbances. In context of other conditions, such as shock (see Chapter 4), lowering of blood pressure is often a late sign of deterioration.

Measuring *urine output* is an essential assessment in a woman who is pregnant or has recently given birth. When there is concern for wellbeing, catheterisation with measurement of hourly urine output is a useful gauge of perfusion, giving valuable information about wellbeing, fluid balance and response to treatment. Optimum urine output is 1 ml/kg/h and the minimal acceptable urine output is 0.5 ml/kg/h. The urine should be tested for proteinuria, infection (leukocytes) and evidence of ketosis.

D: Disability

The midwife will have assessed the level of consciousness when first responding and talking to the woman. A quick method of assessing and documenting the level of consciousness is the AVPU method (see Box 1.4). If the level of consciousness is reduced, a more detailed assessment using the Glasgow Coma Scale (GCS) is indicated. For detailed aspects of neurological response, see Chapter 9. Hypotension and hypoxia may cause confusion and heightened anxiety. Both hyperglycaemia and hypoglycaemia can present as a diminished level of consciousness or changes in behaviour, so the midwife should check the blood sugar as part of the assessment.

Box 1.4 AVPU classification[10]

A: *alert*
V: responds to *voice*
P: responds only to *painful* stimuli
U: *unresponsive* to all stimuli

E: Exposure

Depending on the stage of pregnancy or puerperium, the usual fetal/newborn assessment, antenatal examination or postnatal check should be done. See Box 1.5 for some of the elements of traditional midwifery head-to-toe examination that may be relevant as part of the assessment of a deteriorating condition. Features of infection, blood loss, signs of pre-eclampsia and deteriorating fetal wellbeing will be the most frequent signs the midwife may identify.

Box 1.5 Elements of midwifery head-to-toe examination that may be relevant as part of the assessment of a deteriorating condition

Midwifery antenatal assessment:

- Review medical, obstetric, family and current pregnancy history, estimated date of delivery and gestational age.
- Review general physical and psychological wellbeing.
- Perform abdominal palpation, including symphysis fundal height measurement; enquire regarding fetal movements and fetal heart auscultation/CTG as indicated.
- Examine legs (swelling, pain).
- Enquire regarding any concerns (pain, urine, vaginal loss, headaches, visual disturbances, skin disorders).
- Test BP and urine.
- Review any test results.

Midwifery postnatal assessment:

- Review medical, obstetric, family and current pregnancy history.
- Review labour and delivery details.
- Record and review observations of BP, temperature, pulse and respiratory rate.
- Review general physical and psychological wellbeing.
- Enquire and examine regarding any concerns (breasts, uterine involution, abdominal pain, lochia, wounds, urine and bowels, legs, skin, rashes, any other pain, headaches, visual disturbances).
- Review any test results.

History

As part of the assessment, the midwife will want to find out about the woman's current condition as well as review the notes for factors in her medical, obstetric and family histories that may be relevant. The midwife might ask the woman 'What has bought you to the hospital today?' or an equivalent relevant question such as 'Why are you worried?' (see Box 1.6 for useful questions). The midwife will note the features of her condition and sense of wellbeing that are important to her. Consideration of risk factors, such as prolonged rupture or membranes and the increased risk of sepsis, may give important indicators of the woman's ill health. If the obstetric notes are not available, the midwife will also need to ask about relevant aspects of the pregnancy and birth.

Box 1.6 Useful questions

— How are you?

— What made you come to the hospital today?

— Are you worried about anything?

— How long have you been unwell?

— Do you have any pre-existing illnesses?

— Are you taking any medication? Do you have any allergies?

— Have you taken anything since you became unwell?

— Have you been in contact with anyone with an infective illness?

— Have you got any pain? (see Box 1.2 for useful pain questions)

— Is the baby moving?

Summoning help and ongoing assessment

Modified early obstetric warning system (MEOWS) chart

Assessments of heart and respiratory rate, temperature, blood pressure, level of consciousness and other observations should be recorded on a MEOWS chart and triggers noted. The aim of MEOWS is to identify serious illness early and activate appropriate referral and management. There is currently no standardised MEOWS chart in maternity care. More elaborate tools for risk assessment in relation to PET are being developed,[11] but are based on complex calculations. Electronic bed-side monitoring may give rise to technology-derived 'track and trigger' systems. However, these systems should not replace, but rather supplement, considered, holistic clinical assessment by a midwife standing alongside the woman and responding accordingly.

Getting the correct help in the correct timeframe

The next step of care requires the midwife to summon the correct help in the appropriate timeframe. How to seek help in obstetric emergencies, such as through use of emergency call buttons and dedicated phone numbers, is generally well-rehearsed. In situations that are less urgent but nonetheless need a prompt response, good communication and clear pathways of responsibility are required.

The midwife will normally contact the obstetric and/or anaesthetic lead on call. Details of concerns and medical details will need to be communicated to medical staff in a coherent manner so that they understand the level of deterioration. It is useful for the midwife to relay the information in a structured way using medical language. For example, the midwife may note that a woman doesn't look right. She looks pale and feels clammy and the midwife is concerned. If the midwife rings the doctor and requests an urgent medical review for a woman who looks pale and feels cold, they may not get the required response. However, if the midwife communicates the clinical features – a woman who is Day One post-Caesarean section is tachycardic (90 beats per minute), has increased respirations (22 resps per minute), has oxygen saturation 95% in air, is peripherally shut down, is feeling dizzy, has reduced urine output and does not look well – the doctor is more likely to respond quickly. It is important to remember that the doctor may have to prioritise the demands of a number of clinical situations and the greater detailed clinical information that is communicated will assist this. Box 1.7 gives some pointers with regard to summoning appropriate medical help. Systems such as SBAR (situation, background, assessment, recommendation)[12] or RSVP (reason, story, vital signs, plan)[13] are recommended.

Effective maternity care is delivered by teams rather than individuals. Good teamwork and audit increase the safety of mothers and babies, while poor teamwork, where lessons are not learnt, jeopardises safety.[7] The Kings Fund report 'Safe births – everybody's business'[14] identified that communication between clinicians, particularly at crunch points – such as in referrals between health professionals, during shift changes

---

Box 1.7 Summoning appropriate medical help[15]

- Be familiar with hospital processes for who to call and how.
- Seek help from a senior midwife if appropriate.
- Call the level of obstetric/anaesthetic practitioner appropriate.
- Stand by the phone if possible to respond to bleep call-back.
- Confirm response is from the right person; state the reason for the call and the woman's name and location.
- Have the woman's records and observations to hand.
- Present findings in a structured way, giving only concise relevant details – SBAR or RSVP systems are advocated. Think history, vital signs and conditions and key concerns. What action is required?

and in emergencies – was not always effective. The report recommended that there should be clear and agreed procedures for communication, clarity about team objectives and roles and effective leadership. Good working relationships, respect for others and clear verbal and written communication are essential.

Immediate and ongoing midwifery assessment and care

Oxygen therapy, insertion of wide-bore cannulae, fluid replacement and taking of bloods may form part of the midwife's initial response while waiting for an urgent medical review. Box 1.8 lists actions the midwife may take as part of ongoing assessment and care when a woman is identified with a deteriorating condition. The midwife should also feel able to escalate to a more senior doctor if response is too slow or the condition of the woman warrants it. The frequency of observations needs to be increased with the level of risk. This will aid assessment of the response to any treatment and to note trends.[15]

Box 1.8 Immediate and ongoing midwifery assessment and care[16]

- Seek senior obstetric and anaesthetic review.
- Get senior midwife assistance.
- Maintain assessment of ABCD and respond accordingly if deterioration occurs.
- Increase observation frequency – use automated machine for BP and pulse.
- Apply pulse oximeter and give facial oxygen if required (saturations below 95%, increased respiratory rate, effort).
- Consider optimum position – sitting upright (respiratory symptoms) or lowering head of bed (low blood pressure, feeling faint). If antenatal, tilt the woman at least 15–30 degrees or move onto left side.
- Assess fetal wellbeing. Commence CTG.
- Insert wide-bore cannulae or check IV lines. Take bloods as indicated.
- Catheterise the woman and add hourly urometer if indicated.
- Check medication chart – has any drug been omitted?
- Consider transfer to LW, critical care. Where can she best be assessed? Make arrangements to transfer.
- Check recent lab results and make available for review.
- Prepare equipment – ECG machine, haemacue, arterial blood gas syringes, blood bottles, portable ultrasound machine – as appropriate.
- Maintain contemporaneous notes detailing assessments and plan of care. Commence a more detailed HDU chart.
- Provide sensitive psychological support, explaining the plan of care to the woman and her family.
- Keep communicating with the woman and note any changes.

Further reading

Resuscitation Council (UK). 2017. The ABCDE approach. Available at www.resus.org.uk/resuscitation-guidelines/abcde-approach/. Accessed 9 September 2017.

References

1. Royal College of Anaesthetists (RCOA). 2011. Providing equity of critical and maternity care for the critically ill pregnant or recently pregnant woman. Available at www.rcoa.ac.uk/system/files/CSQ-ProvEqMatCritCare.pdf.
2. National Institute for Health and Care Excellence. 2007. Acutely ill adults in hospital: recognising and responding to deterioration. Clinical guideline 50. Available at www.nice.org.uk/guidance/cg50. Accessed 7 September 2017.
3. Department of Health. 2009. Competencies for recognising and responding to acutely ill patients in hospital. Available at http://webarchive.nationalarchives.gov.uk/2013012319 5821/http://www.dh.gov.uk/en/Publicationsandstatistics/Publications/PublicationsPolicyAnd Guidance/DH_096989. Accessed 9 September 2017.
4. Knight, M, Nair, M, Tuffnell, D, Kenyon, S, Shakespeare, J, Brocklehurst, P and Kurinczuk, JJ (eds) on behalf of MBRRACE-UK. 2016. *Saving lives, improving mothers' care: surveillance of maternal deaths in the UK 2012–2014 and lessons learned to inform maternity care from the UK and Ireland confidential enquiries into maternal deaths and morbidity 2009–2014.* Oxford, UK: National Perinatal Epidemiology Unit, University of Oxford.
5. Centre for Maternal and Child Enquiries (CMACE). 2011. Saving mothers' lives: reviewing maternal deaths to make motherhood safer: 2006–2008. The eighth report on confidential enquiries into maternal deaths in the United Kingdom. *British Journal of Obstetrics and Gynaecology, 118*(1): 1–203.
6. Draycott, T, Sibanda, T, Owen, L, Akande, V, Winter, C, Reading, S and Whitelaw, A. 2006. Does training in obstetric emergencies improve neonatal outcome? *British Journal of Obstetrics and Gynaecology, 113*(2): 177–82.
7. Kirkup, B. 2015. The report of the Morecambe Bay investigation. Available at www.gov.uk/government/publications/morecambe-bay-investigation-report. Accessed 9 September 2017.
8. Royal College of Obstetrics and Gynaecology (RCOG). 2011. Maternal collapse in pregnancy and the puerperium. Green-top guideline No. 56. Available at www.rcog.org.uk/en/guidelines-research-services/guidelines/gtg56/. Accessed 9 September 2017.
9. Jevon, P and Ewens, B. 2012. *Monitoring the critically ill patient.* Oxford, UK: Blackwell Publishing.
10. Resuscitation Council (UK). 2017. The ABCDE approach. Available at www.resus.org.uk/resuscitation-guidelines/abcde-approach/. Accessed 9 September 2017.
11. von Dadelszen, P, Payne, B, Li, J, Ansermino, JM, Broughton Pipkin, F, Côté, AM . . . and Magee, LA. 2011. Prediction of adverse maternal outcomes in pre-eclampsia: development and validation of the full PIERS model. *Lancet, 377*(9761): 219–27. doi: 10.1016/S0140-6736(10)61351-7.
12. NHS institute for innovation and improvement. 2008. SBAR situation–background–assessment–recommendation. Available at http://webarchive.nationalarchives.gov.uk/20110927033236/http://www.institute.nhs.uk/quality_and_service_improvement_tools/quality_and_service_improvement_tools/sbar_-_situation_-_background_-_assessment_-_recommendation.html. Accessed 9 September 2017.
13. Featherstone, P, Chalmers, T and Smith, G. 2008. RSVP: a system for communication of deterioration in hospital patients. *British Journal of Nursing, 17*(13): 860–4.

14. Kings Fund. 2008. Safe births: everybody's business. Available at www.kingsfund.org.uk/sites/default/files/field/field_publication_file/safe-births-everybodys-business-onora-oneill-february-2008.pdf. Accessed 9 September 2017.
15. Dutton, H. 2012. Assessment and recognition of emergencies in acute care. In: Peate, I and Dutton, H (eds). *Acute nursing care: recognising and responding to medical emergencies*. Harlow, UK: Pearson, pp. 1–19.
16. Structured approach to emergencies in the obstetric patient. In: Paterson-Brown, S and Howell, C (eds). 2014. *The MOET course manual: managing obstetric emergencies and trauma*. Cambridge, UK: Cambridge University Press, pp. 17–21.

Chapter 2

Haemodynamic monitoring

Introduction

Ongoing assessment is central to the care of those who are critically ill, and haemo-dynamic assessment is concerned with all the observations necessary to evaluate the cardiovascular function of the woman. However, interpretation of haemodynamic data must be combined not only with frequent clinical assessment but also with effective clinical treatment.[1] Haemodynamic monitoring can help to determine the diagnosis, indicate the appropriate therapy and monitor the response to the therapy.[2]

Haemodynamic assessment can include non-invasive and invasive techniques. It is also important to note that the midwife undertaking these assessments will be evaluating other significant indicators, such as level of consciousness, mood state and various physical signs such as skin temperature or condition. All these findings feed into the overall evaluation of the woman, ensuring an accurate assessment that may pick up subtle signs of deterioration before more major ones are obvious. Early recog-nition and prompt treatment are likely to improve the outcome.

Methods of non-invasive haemodynamic monitoring

Respiratory assessment

The respiratory rate and quality is considered to be an early indicator of cellular dysfunction. The rate and depth of respirations will initially increase in response to cellular hypoxia.[2] Respiratory assessment should be unobtrusive and include rate, depth, regularity and sound.[3]

The respiratory rate should be counted over a full minute, as critically ill women may have irregular or laboured breathing. Influences on the rate may be recent physical activity or the presence of pain. For detailed assessment of the respiratory system, see Chapter 7.

A normal respiratory rate is usually between 12 and 20, with tachypnoea considered to be > 18/20 and bradypnoea < 12, although there are a variety of parameters quoted in the literature that are considered normal for childbearing women. There needs to be careful documentation on a MEOWS chart, as the trend may be significant.

Pulse oximetry

Pulse oximetry (oxygen 'saturations' or 'sats') is frequently used along with respiratory assessment. It measures the percentage of oxygen-saturation of haemoglobin in the circulation, not the quantity of haemoglobin or the oxygen available. Therefore, saturation readings should always be interpreted in relation to haemoglobin levels,[4] as a woman may have normal saturations but still be hypoxic.[5] However, pulse oximetry can provide a useful continuous view of trends and responses to (or need for) oxygen therapy, and can act as an indicator of a deterioration in condition.[2]

The saturation probe is usually positioned on a finger, toe or earlobe, and should be changed every 4 hours[6] as there is a potential for burns, especially if the woman has a vulnerable circulatory status or skin integrity.

Red and infrared wavelengths of light are passed through the peripheral tissue. The 'redness' of the saturated haemoglobin absorbs the light and is converted into a percentage.[7] The light should pass from the top to the bottom of the limb (check light direction before applying the monitor).[3] A normal reading is considered to be > 95%.

The accuracy depends on the flow of blood through the light being adequate, and this may be compromised by poor circulation (including following a large blood loss), movement such as shivering, dark nail polish, false nails or a poorly-fitted probe (too much extraneous light).[3]

Peripheral pulse

The pulse is a rhythmic wave of pressure or distention transmitted along elastic arterial walls in response to systolic contraction of the heart. In hospital situations, the pulse rate is commonly monitored by various machines; the number they register may be useful (although it is not always accurate), but taking a pulse manually produces much valuable information.

A pulse can be felt wherever the artery can be palpated against something firm, usually bone. Common sites for manual assessment of pulse include the radial, carotid, femoral and brachial arteries. The pulse can also be heard with a stethoscope and should be assessed for rate, rhythm and volume.

- **Rate:** tachycardia is considered to be > 90, and bradycardia < 60. A rising pulse rate as well as a persistent tachycardia is an abnormal sign, warranting further investigation.
- **Rhythm:** an irregular rhythm may indicate an underlying cardiac dysfunction or electrolyte imbalance, and an ECG may be needed.[2] A mild cardiac arrhythmia (e.g. extra beats) may be harmless, but should always be assessed[3] (see Chapter 8).

- **Volume:** the amplitude of the pulse is a reflection of strength and elasticity of the arterial walls. Weak – or thready – and rapid is a characteristic sign of hypovolaemia.[8] A full, bounding or throbbing pulse can indicate changes in the amount of blood being pumped, and may be indicative of heart block, heart failure or early stages of septic shock.[2]

Pulse rates can be influenced by many situations common in childbirth; for example, anaemia from blood loss, certain medications and excitement. However, less benign reasons could be infection (even without fever), ongoing haemorrhage or fluid and/or electrolyte imbalance, including dehydration or disease.[3]

When a sustained pulse rate of more than 90 is present, a cause should always be established. For example, a woman who has recently given birth, with a blood loss resulting in a postnatal haemoglobin of 90 g/l, may have been assessed and prescribed iron tablets but still initially have a raised pulse. This should be monitored to ensure it does not continue to rise, and causes other than mild anaemia need to be excluded.

Skin assessment and capillary refill

Much useful information can be received by simply observing and touching the woman during specific assessments or routine care.

Observation of the peripheries can assess colour and warmth. Mottled/pale, cold and/or clammy peripheries may indicate poor perfusion[4] (although causes can be varied), whereas abnormal warmth and/or flushing may indicate excessive dilation, perhaps caused by sepsis. Examination may also reveal oedema, ulceration or other symptoms of potential haemodynamic compromise.[9]

A capillary refill test is frequently done to assess the adequacy of the peripheral perfusion,[10] although, in pregnancy, oedema may complicate this.[11] The woman's hand is elevated to the level of her heart (or slightly higher) and her fingernail or fingertip is pressed on for 5 seconds. The blanching should disappear within 2 seconds of release.[9] Normal is < 2 seconds,[12] and a delayed response (> 2 seconds) suggests poor peripheral perfusion, although this could be influenced by extraneous conditions such as cold ambient temperature or poor lighting.[2]

Temperature

There are many forms of temperature-measuring devices available. Measurement of core temperature is seen as the most important, but none of the core sites (cranium, thoracic and abdominal cavities) can be accessed non-invasively, so measurements obtained via the ear, forehead, mouth, axilla or rectum are commonly used.

Tympanic thermometers are theoretically the most accurate, as the carotid artery supplies the tympanic membrane as well as the nearby hypothalamus.[13] Disposable chemical thermometers are often used for axillary measurement – however, as they depend on visual interpretation and have a limited range, their accuracy may not be optimal.[4]

An increased temperature is considered to be the first indicator of infection or sepsis. However, it must be remembered that pyrexia is a symptom, not a disease, and may be metabolic or infective in origin. Anti-pyrexial medication (for example, paracetamol) is widely used, and, when assessing temperature, it must be checked that the woman has not taken any drugs that may influence the accuracy of the recording.

Blood pressure (non-invasive)

Blood pressure (BP) is the force exerted by the circulating volume of blood on the walls of the arteries. Changes in cardiac output or peripheral resistance can affect the BP; for example, a woman with a low cardiac output may be able to maintain her blood pressure by vasoconstricting, whereas a woman who is vasodilated (e.g., as a result of sepsis) may be hypotensive despite a high cardiac output.

Blood pressure assessment allows evaluation of the cardiovascular status. It is an assessment of particular importance in pregnancy, and it has been identified that a woman with a BP greater than 150/100 should be receiving treatment, and a reading of > 180 systolic should be considered a medical emergency.[14] For the woman to receive appropriate and timely care, assessment of her blood pressure must be accurate.

Blood pressure measurements in the UK are done either via automated oscillatory machines or auscultatory manual machines. Potential influences on the accuracy of BP recordings are found in Box 2.1.

- Auscultatory machines ('manual') use a sphygmomanometer: a cuff with a rubber bladder within, inflating bulb, manometer and control valve. It may be mercury or anaeroid. The Korotkoff sounds are identified through a stethoscope: K1 (clear tapping audible) for systolic and K5 (disappearance of sound) for diastolic.
- Automated oscillatory BP machines allow an automatic inflation of the cuff (until all oscillations caused by arterial pulsations are extinguished), which then deflates, identifying alteration in oscillatory amplitude, transducing into mean systolic and diastolic pressures and displaying this information onto a screen.[4]

MAP (mean arterial pressure) is calculated by most automated BP machines, although a formula can also be applied to manual readings to obtain this. It averages the pressure across the whole pulse cycle, and is considered to provide a more valuable assessment of perfusion. This may be particularly useful in hypotension.[15]

Box 2.1 Influences on accuracy of BP measurement

— Size of cuff: the cuff should cover 80% of the circumference of the woman's upper arm.[16] Too-small cuffs will over-read.[4]

— Upper arm at heart level: if the arm is positioned lower than heart level, the reading can be abnormally high,[17] and if the arm is above heart level, an incorrect low reading may result.[18]

— Smoking, eating, talking and exercise will increase blood pressure.[19]

— 'White coat syndrome' is when a woman may exhibit an above normal blood pressure reading in a clinical setting, but not at other times.[20]

Methods of invasive haemodynamic monitoring

Invasive haemodynamic monitoring can provide an in-depth assessment of a woman's cardiovascular status to inform clinical decisions and guide and evaluate treatments and interventions. The most commonly-used pieces of equipment of this sort overseen by midwives in UK maternity units are arterial lines and CVP (central venous pressure) lines.

Both arterial lines and CVP lines have transducers to enable the pressure readings to be displayed on a monitor. To maintain the patency of the cannula and tubing and prevent back-flow of blood, a bag of (0.9%) saline should be connected to the transducer tubing and kept under continuous pressure, thereby facilitating a continuous flush.[2] When caring for transducers, the best practice, at a minimum of once each shift, will include:

- checking cannula site(s);
- checking the flush bag;
- ensuring the pressure bag remains inflated to ensure continuous flushing;
- checking all connections to make sure none are becoming loose.

Invasive arterial pressure monitoring (or intra-arterial measurement)

An arterial line is valuable as it allows dynamic beat-to-beat monitoring of the systemic circulation, providing information on respiratory and metabolic function. The continuous intra-arterial pressure provides more frequent, accurate data than auscultating peripheral BPs.[21] The advantage of an arterial line is the continuous visual display of both the arterial blood pressure and the arterial pressure waveform. There is also easy (and non-painful) access to arterial blood for sampling.

An arterial line consists of a cannula that is inserted into an artery and connected to a sterile system, which is primed with heparinised saline and fitted to a transducer. The pulsations produced will reverberate against the membrane in the transducer, and be displayed on a monitor in both a waveform and a digital reading.[22] When initially set up, the system must be calibrated.

The insertion sites for an arterial line may include the radial, brachial, dorsalis pedis or femoral arteries, but the radial artery is the commonest for ease of observation, and, because this artery is close to the surface, it can be visualised more easily. If the woman is very hypotensive, the femoral artery may be used, but this is unlikely in a maternity setting. Figure 2.1 illustrates the normal arterial line waveform. Features to note include:

- The area under the wave indicates pulse volume.
- The upstroke indicates myocardial contractility (normal should be almost vertical; shallower upstrokes indicate poor flow).
- The highest point of the waveform corresponds to the systolic pressure.
- The downstrokes are normally almost vertical; gentler downslopes occur with vasoconstriction.
- A dicrotic notch appears when the aortic valve closes.
- The lowest point or baseline is the diastolic pressure.

To ensure an accurate BP, an accurate waveform is necessary. See Box 2.2 for troubleshooting suggestions if the trace is flat.

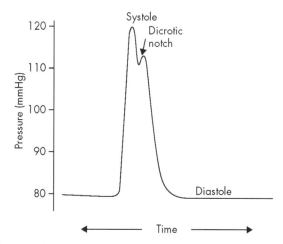

Figure 2.1 Arterial line waveform

Source: Philip Woodrow. 2012. *Intensive care nursing*, 3rd edition. Oxford, UK: Routledge.

Box 2.2 Troubleshooting suggestions when the arterial waveform looks inaccurate

- Check the woman's wellbeing;
- Check the proximal join, as the cannula may be kinked or compressed against the vessel wall;
- Check the circuit for air-bubbles;
- Check the circuit connections;
- Check that the tubing in the circuit is not kinked;
- Check that the flush bag has adequate fluid and sufficient pressure is being maintained;
- Check patency by withdrawing blood;
- Check the BP manually.

However, it must be remembered when caring for a woman with an arterial line that she will require very close supervision, partly because her condition is likely to be unstable or she would not have needed this intervention, but also because if the arterial line itself becomes disconnected, massive haemorrhage can occur.[22] Complications can occur during insertion of the arterial line, or a time following, and the midwife must ensure constant observation is made for these:

1. No drugs should be given through arterial lines, so careful identification and labelling[23] of the line is necessary.

2. There is a great potential for massive haemorrhage if the patency of the system is breached. A well-secured transparent dressing should cover the cannula, so the site can be easily observed. The limb should be exposed (not covered by bedlinen) and constantly observed for signs of decrease in perfusion and disconnection of the cannula.[24] Routine checks should be made of the system to ensure that no connections are becoming loose and all three-way taps are kept closed. Monitor alarms should be set.

3. Women with an arterial line are by definition susceptible to infection, as it is expected that their condition is vulnerable, and therefore screening for infection needs to be frequent.

4. Other, less-common complications include arterial occlusion, thrombosis/embolisation, aneurysm, haematoma and ischaemia distal to the cannula, causing tissue necrosis and air embolus (see Box 2.3). A specific condition of retrograde embolisation, where small blood clots may form either within the catheter or at the tip (which if flushed into the systemic system may affect circulation), can be screened for by the midwife. Signs would be discolouration, mottling, coolness or altered sensation, plus compromised pulses both proximal and distal to catheter insertion.[24]

Box 2.3 Air embolism

An air embolism is a rare but potentially fatal occurrence. It is most commonly associated with central line catheters (where the incidence has been suggested to be 0.2%–1%),[25] but is also associated with haemodialysis, trauma and childbirth.[26] 50–100 ml may be fatal.[27] If suspected, diagnosis is difficult but it may be seen on a chest X-ray or Doppler ultrasound. A transoesophageal echocardiograph may also be used.

Central venous pressure (CVP) monitoring

The CVP line is generally used for monitoring and access. It is considered helpful in the assessment of cardiac function, circulating blood volume, vascular tone and response to treatment.[2] The CVP measurement reflects the filling pressure (or preload) to the right side of the heart and assists assessment of intraventricular volume and right-sided heart function.[28] It may indicate the blood volume, as it reflects the pressure within the great veins (which hold 60% of total blood volume), and it may help to avoid either under-transfusion or fluid overload by assessing blood volume deficits.[3]

The CVP line can also be used for rapid fluid resuscitation, drug and fluid administration – in particular when there is poor venous access – and parenteral nutrition.[22]

Readings are dependent on cardiac function, intravascular volume, vascular tone, intrinsic venous tone, increased intra-abdominal/intrathoracic pressure and vasopressor therapy. A trend of readings is usually necessary, as an isolated measurement can be misleading.

The CVP line is a hollow radiopaque cannula, which is inserted percutaneously so that the tip lies either in the superior vena cava or within the right atrium of the heart.

There are two methods of measurement:

- The manometer system, measured by a manual water column that is inserted into an IV set, producing intermittent readings. This is rarely used today.
- The transducer system, where the line is connected to a transducer system and will display continuous readings on a monitor.

When setting up a CVP, calibration of the system according to the manufacturer's recommendations is necessary. Although this is frequently done when initially sited by the anaesthetist, the midwife needs to be able to do this, as recalibration may be necessary during the time the midwife is caring for this woman.

The transducer is zeroed at approximately the level of the woman's heart and the flush bag is maintained at an adequate pressure (usually 300 mmHg) to avoid back-flow. A heparin flush is not usually necessary. Careful capping of three-way taps is vital to avoid air embolus.

The most common site for the CVP insertion is via the internal jugular vein or from a peripheral vein in the arm with a longer catheter. This approach is preferred when DIC is present, as there is less risk of bleeding at the insertion. The catheter is inserted under strict asepsis, followed by correct placement being confirmed, usually by X-ray. The catheter is sutured in place with a sterile dressing applied, and is then connected to the primed monitoring system.[22]

The secure transparent dressing over the site will allow for observation. Infection from CVPs is high (~ 4–18%),[2] so there must be strict asepsis during the initial insertion and whenever taking samples, giving drugs or changing the dressing. Changing lines and dressings is done according to local guidelines – if clean and intact, the dressing may only be changed every seven days.[4] After removal of the CVP, it is common to culture the tip.

The CVP line may consist of one, three, four or five lumina. A single lumen catheter is used in the arm and multi-lumen in the internal jugular or subclavian veins. The individual lumina are usually labelled separately with their use for regular drugs or fluids. If not in use, cannulae may need to be flushed regularly. An infusion with drugs should be through a separate dedicated lumen, as a 'flush' could cause a sudden surge in drug administration

It is vital that inspection is made regularly to ensure connections are secure enough to prevent exsanguination, infection and air embolus. Midwives will probably have local guidelines to follow to ensure this is done.

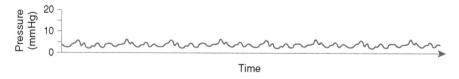

Figure 2.2 CVP line waveform

Source: Tina Moore and Philip Woodrow (eds). 2009. *High dependency nursing care*, 2nd edition. Oxford, UK: Routledge.

The CVP trace on the monitor is a slightly undulating waveform, which reflects the changes in the right atrial pressure during the cardiac cycle.[2]

The normal range of CVP readings are 3–10 mmHg (5–12 cmH$_2$O if a water manometer is being used). The wide variety means that emphasis should be placed on dynamic change over time. Trends are more significant than an absolute figure.

- A *low* CVP reading usually indicates fluid loss, hypovolaemia or dehydration.
- A *high* CVP reading may indicate hypervolaemia, cardiac failure, pulmonary embolism, increased intrathoracic pressure, cardiac tamponade, high blood viscosity or fluid overload. A very high reading may result from pulmonary oedema.[4] If the woman is in respiratory distress, measurements should be taken at the end of expiration, as the CVP will be artificially higher because of positive intrathoracic pressure.[29]

Box 2.4 Troubleshooting suggestions when the CVP waveform looks inaccurate

— A persistently high reading with a dampened trace could be caused by an occluded catheter.

— A falsely high measurement is possible if infusions continue to be administered through the CVP – infusions should be temporarily switched off while CVP measurement is taken.

Local or systemic infection is the most common complication of CVP monitoring.[30] Others include:

- thrombus formation at either the tip of the catheter or its surround (may be prevented by regular flushing with normal saline);
- air emboli (see Box 2.3);
- pneumothorax;
- haemothorax;
- cardiac tamponade;
- cardiac arrhythmias;
- pain;
- haemorrhage;
- insertion accidents (puncture of surrounding tissues or malposition of the catheter).

When removing CVP lines, women should be positioned flat or head-down, to avoid air emboli. Women should be asked to breathe out and hold their breath during removal so intrathoracic pressure equals atmospheric pressure.[4] Direct pressure on the site after removal for at least 5 minutes,[22] plus care in maintaining closed caps throughout the system, will also help to avoid air emboli.

Other methods of haemodynamic assessment

X-ray

A chest X-ray will provide valuable information for respiratory assessment, as it will show the lungs, heart and major blood vessels, revealing any abnormalities of the chest. Chest X-rays are not contraindicated in pregnancy, although shielding of the uterus is still advised. Women may be concerned about having an X-ray and midwives can provide reassurance regarding the safety of a normal chest X-ray.[31]

Ultrasound scan (USS)

Besides visualisation of any area of concern, USS may also aid cardiac investigations. It may also be used for fetal assessment, especially growth, liquor volume estimation and Doppler studies to underpin timing for delivery, or because signs of fetal deterioration often precede a change in maternal condition.

Transthoracic echocardiography

This is a non-invasive method of measuring cardiac structure and function. It is primarily used after a myocardial infarction (MI), but it can also form part of a more general haemodynamic assessment. Echocardiograms can be considered relatively accessible, as testing can often be done at the bedside.[2] (See also Chapter 8.)

Transoesophageal echocardiography

An ultrasound technique that involves introducing a scope-like probe on the end of a flexible gastroscope-like probe, which can be manoeuvred within the oesophagus and stomach, close to the heart, to measure cardiac structure and function. (See also Chapter 8.)

MRI (magnetic resonance imaging)

MRI is a technique used in radiology to form pictures of the anatomy and the physiological processes of the body. MRI scanners use strong magnetic fields, radio waves and field gradients to generate images of the organs in the body. Although safety during pregnancy has not yet been totally established, no harmful effects on the fetus have been reported.[32] However, imaging should be avoided during the first trimester if possible.[33]

CT (computed tomography)

A computed tomography (CT) is a diagnostic imaging tool that uses X-ray beams in multiple directions, creating image slices that can be used to reconstruct two-dimensional and three-dimensional images. Safety issues vary with gestation and current recommendations are for use only when benefits clearly outweigh potential risks.[32]

Pulmonary artery pressure monitoring

This is also known as a Swan Ganz and is a multi-lumen directional flow catheter.[2] It is used to evaluate cardiac function and detect problems in the pulmonary vasculature, underpinning decisions to optimise cardiac output and delivery of oxygen while minimising risk of pulmonary oedema. This is unlikely to be used in maternity critical care units, but will be seen in general ICU and coronary care areas.

References

1. Sturgess, D and Morgan, TJ. 2009. Haemodynamic monitoring. In: Bersten, A and Soni, N (eds). *Oh's intensive care manual*. Philadelphia, PA: Butterworth Heinemann Elsevier, pp. 105–22.
2. Jevon, P and Ewens, B. 2012. *Monitoring the critically ill patient*. Oxford, UK: Blackwell Publishing.
3. Johnson, R and Taylor, W. 2016. *Skills for midwifery practice*. Edinburgh, UK: Elsevier.
4. Woodrow, P. 2012. *Intensive care nursing*. London: Routledge.
5. Higgins, D. 2005. Pulse oximetry. *Nursing Times*, *101*(6): 34.
6. MDA (Medical Devices Agency). March 2001. Tissue necrosis caused by pulse oximeter probes: safety notice MDA SN 2001(08). London: Medical Devices Agency.
7. Chandler, T. 2000. Oxygen saturation monitoring. *Paediatric Nursing*, *12*(8): 37–42.
8. Bickley, L. 2016. *Bates' guide to physical examination and history taking*. Philadelphia, PA: Lippincott, Williams & Wilkins.
9. Moore, T and Woodrow, P. 2009. High dependency nursing care: observation, intervention and support for Level 2 patients. London: Routledge.
10. Nathan, H, El Ayadi, A, Hezelgrave, NL, Seed, P, Butrick, E, Miller, S . . . and Shennan, AH. 2015. Shock index: an effective predictor of outcome in postpartum haemorrhage? *BJOC*, *122*(2): 268–75.
11. Nihoyannopoulus, P. 2007. Cardiovascular examination in pregnancy and the approach to the diagnosis of cardiac disorder. In: Oakley, C and Warnes, C (eds). *Heart disease in pregnancy*. Oxford, UK: BMJ Publishing/Blackwell, pp. 18–28.
12. Gwinnutt, M and Gwinnutt, C. 2016. *Lecture notes clinical anaesthesia*. Oxford, UK: Wiley-Blackwell.
13. Stanhope, N. 2006. Temperature measurement in the Phase 1 PACU. *Journal of PeriAnesthesia Nursing*, *21*(1): 27–36.
14. Centre for Maternal and Child Enquiries (CMACE). 2011. Saving mothers' lives: reviewing maternal deaths to make motherhood safer: 2006–2008. The eighth report on confidential enquiries into maternal deaths in the United Kingdom. *British Journal of Obstetrics and Gynaecology*, *118*(1): s1–203.
15. Woodrow, P. 2016. *Nursing acutely ill adults*. Abingdon, UK: Routledge.
16. British Hypertensive Society. 2015. *Blood pressure measurement* (website). Available at http://bhsoc.org/files/9013/4390/7747/BP_Measurement_Poster_-_Manual.pdf. Accessed 21 September 2017.
17. Dougherty, L and Lister, S. 2008. *The Royal Marsden Hospital manual of clinical nursing procedures*. Chichester, UK: Wiley-Blackwell.
18. Beevers, G, Lip, G and O'Brien, E. 2001. Blood pressure measurement. Part 1, sphygmomanometry: factors common to all techniques. *British Medical Journal*, *322*(7292): 981–5.
19. Bothamley, J and Boyle, M. 2008. How to measure blood pressure. *Midwives*, *11*(1): 29.
20. Verdecchia, P, Staessen, J, White, W, Imai, Y and O'Brien, E. 2002. Properly defining white coat hypertension. *European Heart Journal*, *23*(2): 106–9.

21. Marshall, J and Raynor, M (eds). 2010. *Advancing skills in midwifery practice*. Edinburgh, UK: Churchill Livingstone.

22. Billington, M and Stevenson, M. 2007. *Critical care in childbearing for midwives*. Oxford, UK: Blackwell Publishing.

23. NPSA (National Patient Safety Agency). 2008. *Problems with infusions and sampling from arterial lines*. London: NPSA.

24. Garretson, S. 2005. Haemodynamic monitoring: arterial catheterization. *Nursing Standard*, *19*(31): 55–64.

25. Gordy, S and Rowell, S. 2013. Vascular air embolism. *International Journal of Critical Illness and Injury Science*, *3*(1): 73–6.

26. Mirski, M, Lele, A, Fitzsimmons, L and Toung, TJ. 2007. Diagnosis and treatment of vascular air embolism. *Anesthesiology*, *106*(1): 164–77.

27. Polderman, K and Girbes, A. 2002. Central venous catheter use. Part 1: mechanical complications. *Intensive Care Medicine*, *28*(1): 1–17.

28. McGee, W, Headley, J and Frazier, J. 2009. *Quick guide to cardiopulmonary care*. Irvine, CA: Edwards Critical Care Education.

29. Kent, B and Dowd, B. 2007. Assessment, monitoring and diagnostics. In Elliott, D, Aitken, L and Chaboyer, W (eds). *ACCCN's critical care nursing*. Marrickville: Mosby Elsevier.

30. Cole, E. 2007. Measuring CVP. *Nursing Standard*, *22*(7): 40–2.

31. Annamraju, H and Mackillop, L. 2017. Respiratory disease in pregnancy. *Obstetrics, Gynaecology and Reproductive Medicine*, *27*(4): 105–11.

32. Waksmonski, C. 2014. Cardiac imaging and functional assessment in pregnancy. *Seminars in Perinatology*, *38*(5): 240–4.

33. Regitz-Zagrosek, V, Lundqvist, CB, Borghi, C, Cifkova, R, Ferreira, R, Foidart, J-M . . . and Torracca, L on behalf of the European Society of Gynecology (ESG), the Association for European Paediatric Cardiology (AEPC) and the German Society for Gender Medicine (DgesGM). 2011. Guidelines on the management of cardiovascular diseases during pregnancy: the task force on the management of cardiovascular diseases during pregnancy of the European Society of Cardiology (ECS). *European Heart Journal*, *32*: 3147–97.

Chapter 3

Fluid balance, electrolytes and fluid replacement

Introduction

Accurate measurement of fluid intake and output is an important part of the assessment of women who are unwell, and yet it is frequently observed that records of fluid balance are incomplete, confusing or difficult to maintain accurately.[1] The physiological changes in pregnancy – plasma expansion and increased colloid osmotic pressure – alter normal homeostatic mechanisms. Conditions such as postpartum haemorrhage (PPH) and pre-eclampsia (PET) can cause significant disruption to normal fluid balance. The unreliability of estimations of blood loss in PPH, and concealed bleeding (post-surgery, antepartum haemorrhage (APH)) can lead to unrecognised fluid deficit and hypovolaemic shock. The danger of fluid overload as a cause of maternal death from pulmonary oedema in women with pre-eclampsia is well-documented.[2,3,4]

Midwives are commonly required to administer IV fluids and blood transfusions, monitor urine output and maintain records of fluid balance. The midwife needs to understand when and why fluids are needed and what fluid replacement is aiming to achieve, and be able to assess the effectiveness of fluid administration.

Physiology

Body fluids are dilute solutions of water and electrolytes. Fluid balance is the assessment of the volume of water lost from the body and the volume of water gained. Optimum fluid balance will achieve a normal and consistent circulating blood volume with sufficient pressure to deliver oxygen and nutrients to the cells. The body aims to maintain adequate blood volume by a variety of hormonal mechanisms, central nervous system (CNS) responses, regulation of the renal system and control by the adrenal cortex.

Fluid compartments

Most body fluid (around 66% of total fluid volume) is held within the cell (intracellular fluid (ICF)). The rest is outside the cell (extracellular fluid (ECF)). ECF is contained either within the blood vessels, predominantly as the main component of blood plasma, or in the gaps between cells, known as the interstitial space (see Figure 3.1). During pregnancy, there is a 40% increase in circulating blood volume.

Although these compartments are classified as separate areas, water and electrolytes continually circulate between them. Body water contains dissolved electrolytes including sodium (Na), potassium (K), chloride, bicarbonate, calcium and magnesium.

The ICF is separated from the ECF by two specific membranes:

1. The *capillary membrane* is a very thin semi-permeable membrane that covers a large surface area. It is designed to facilitate the exchange of fluids and nutrients between the plasma and interstitial fluid.[1] While it is very thin and allows most molecules within the plasma to filter through, plasma proteins and red blood cells are too large to cross.[1,5] Water moves freely between the capillary vessel and the interstitial compartment by osmosis, and electrolytes move from an area of high concentration to one of low concentration by diffusion.
2. The interstitial compartment and the fluid in cells are separated by specialised cell layers. Many important solutes are transported actively across *cell membranes*, including sodium, potassium, hydrogen ions and glucose.[6]

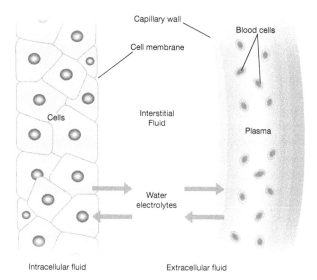

Figure 3.1 Fluid compartments

Fluid movement between compartments

Normal movement of fluids between blood and tissues depends upon two forces, and works like a 'push' and 'pull' mechanism.[6] *Hydrostatic pressure* is the 'pushing' force, determined by the pumping action of the heart and blood pressure, which forces fluid and solutes through the fine capillary walls into the interstitial fluid. *Osmotic pressure*

is the 'pulling' force, which is mainly determined by the concentration of protein molecules acting like a magnet, attracting water and keeping it within the blood vessel.
This is known as colloid osmotic pressure. Pressure created by the concentration of
electrolytes is called crystalloid oncotic pressure.[5,6]

Oxygenated blood arrives at the arterial end of the capillary. The pressure here
(around 32 mmHg) is greater than the colloid oncotic pressure of the interstitial fluid,
and therefore fluid containing oxygen and nutrients is pushed out of the capillary into
the interstitial compartment. At the venous end, colloid oncotic pressure in the vessels
is greater (the protein concentration has increased as fluid has moved out but proteins
have not) and hydrostatic pressure is lower (12 mmHg), so fluid containing carbon
dioxide and wastes is drawn back into the blood vessels.[5] Some excess fluid is drained
into the lymphatic system. The interstitial fluid therefore has a role in maintaining
sufficient blood pressure. When there is excess interstitial fluid, this is noted as
oedema of the tissues. The physiological changes of pregnancy cause a reduction in
the colloid oncotic pressure in blood vessels due to plasma volume expansion thereby
reducing the concentration of protein in blood overall. This explains the tendency
towards dependent oedema in the feet and ankles, commonly seen in pregnant women.

Physiological controls of fluid in the body

The predominant control of fluid balance is regulation of the urine output, controlled
by the kidneys.

Table 3.1 gives a summary of the hormone controls of fluid balance.

Table 3.1 Hormone controls of fluid balance

Location	Hormone	Action
Central nervous system (CNS) Osmoreceptors		Specialised brain cells that stimulate thirst and thus the need to drink Trigger the release of *antidiuretic hormone* (ADH)
Produced in the hypothalamus and stored in the posterior pituitary	Antidiuretic hormone (ADH)	As the name implies, ADH reduces fluid loss by acting on the kidney to produce less urine that is more concentrated
Renin–angiotensin–aldosterone system		
Kidney	Renin	The kidney detects a reduction in blood volume and produces the enzyme *renin*; renin leads to the release of *angiotensinogen*
Liver	Angiotensinogen	Produced by liver cells and converted in the plasma into *angiotensin 1*
Plasma	Angiotensin 1	Converted in the lungs into *angiotensin 2*
Lungs	Angiotensin 2: a very powerful vasopressor	Causes vasoconstriction of the arterioles of the kidney, leading to reduced glomerular filtration rate; angiotensin 2 also acts on the adrenal cortex to produce *aldosterone*
Adrenal cortex	Aldosterone	Increases the reabsorption of sodium in the nephron, which pulls water with it

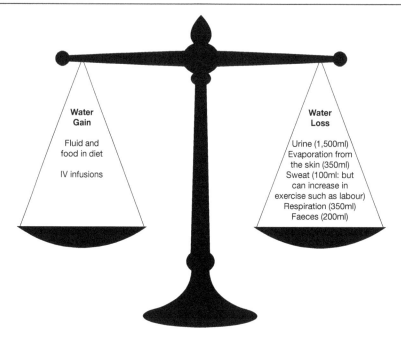

Figure 3.2 Fluid balance

Fluid balance

In simple terms, assessment and recording of fluid balance by measuring what goes in (oral fluid, IV fluids) and what comes out (urine, blood loss) should be straightforward (see Figure 3.2). However, it is common to observe records of fluid balance that are inaccurate and thus may have limited value in determining the management of care. Inaccurate estimation of blood loss, poor recordings such as 'out to toilet', omitting fluids associated with drug administration and incorrect calculations of cumulative amounts are examples of problems associated with keeping accurate fluid balance.

Fluid balance charts

The aim of a fluid balance chart is to keep an accurate record of the woman's fluid input and output to facilitate recognition of irregularities. See Box 3.1 for examples of when a fluid balance chart should be used.

The output side should document all measurable fluid loss, which will predominantly be urine output, estimated blood loss and vomit, but may include fluid from a nasogastric tube and loss from drains. Hourly urine measurement is most informative and use of a urometer is advocated when the woman is unwell. Urine output that stops suddenly is commonly due to kinked or blocked catheter tubing, which needs to be corrected. Input will include IV infusions, fluid taken orally, blood and blood products and fluids used as part of medication administration. Volumetric pumps are often used to aid measured delivery of IV fluids.

The midwife should be mindful of insensible fluid loss that cannot be measured. Examples of insensible fluid loss include evaporation/sweating (around 450 ml daily),

---

Box 3.1 Indications for a fluid balance chart

- Following any haemorrhage;
- IV infusion;
- Post-surgery;
- Pre-eclampsia;

- Medical conditions such renal disease, cardiac disorders and diabetes;
- When catheterised;
- Vomiting or diarrhoea;
- Sepsis.

---

and this loss will rise when the woman has a high temperature. A higher respiratory rate will increase fluid loss (around 500 ml daily in normal respiratory rate) and excessive exercise (such as in labour) will exacerbate fluid loss.

It is recommended that fluid balance be written on a single 24-hour sheet and that charts are calculated from the same time. The recording of fluid balance should commence at any time – for example, at the point a catheter is inserted. However, to record 24-hour balance, a new chart is started at a designated time within an organisation (for example, 8 a.m. each day). To improve accuracy, it is important to measure volumes where possible. Include records of blood loss and fluid administration in theatre to make post-operative records more meaningful. Weigh blood loss to improve accuracy. Give the woman a jug for urine. Know what volume is in a standard glass.

In the critical care setting, fluid balance should ideally be recorded on the daily care record charts (sometimes called HDU or ICU charts). These charts combine records of fluid input and output alongside observations, treatment regimens and staff comments. Having care interventions alongside records of assessment enables the effectiveness of treatment to be determined and reduces the possibility of events being overlooked.[7]

Disruptions to fluid balance

Increased fluid loss can be caused by haemorrhage, conditions causing high temperature, raised respiratory rate, diarrhoea, vomiting and polyuria associated with diabetes. Increased exercise, such as in labour, increases insensible loss. The woman may not be eating and drinking as normal or be kept intentionally nil-by-mouth for surgical or medical reasons. Medications such as hydralazine and epidural medication can cause a reduction in blood pressure and may require a pre-load of fluid to compensate for this.

In maternity care, *fluid overload* is most likely to occur in cases of pre-eclampsia. When there is excess interstitial fluid, perhaps as a complication of pre-eclampsia, pregnant women can develop dangerous pulmonary oedema in lung tissue, which interferes with adequate oxygenation (see Chapter 7). Compensatory mechanisms to fluid loss involve the kidneys retaining fluid by concentrating urine and movement of fluid from interstitial compartment back into vessels to initially maintain blood pressure. However, once the interstitial space becomes depleted, blood pressure drops, the pulse becomes thready and weak, the peripheries shut down, the skin feels cool to the touch and urine output falls.

Some women with renal dysfunction can present with polyuria as their condition worsens. See Table 3.2 for a list of conditions that contribute to fluid imbalance in maternity care

Table 3.2 Conditions that contribute to fluid imbalance in maternity care

Hypovolaemic shock	Large amount of blood leaves the vascular space, as seen in PPH.
Pre-eclampsia (PET)	Reduced glomerular filtration and damage to endothelial lining of glomerulus lead to reduced urine output and increased protein loss; colloid oncotic pressure is affected by the protein loss and fluid is pulled into the interstitial space; erroneous over-administration of IV fluids can push more fluid into the interstitial compartment, which can result in life-threatening pulmonary oedema.
Septic shock	Release of cytokines causes vasodilation and increased capillary permeability; this allows water and large molecules to move into the interstitial space, resulting in loss of protein, hypovolaemia and interstitial oedema.
Anaphylactic shock	Anaphylactic shock involves mast cell degranulation releasing histamine, bradykinin and other vasoactive substances; this causes fluid to move from the blood vessels into the interstitial space, causing a reduction in blood pressure and tissue hypoxia.
Hyperglycaemia	In untreated or inadequately-treated diabetes, glycosuria increases fluid loss, increasing urine output.

Assessment of fluid and electrolyte status

Assessment of fluid and electrolyte status will involve:

- assessment for any obvious bleeding (see Chapter 5);
- clinical assessment following an ABCDE-structured approach;
- review of fluid balance charts, in particular a review of urine output;
- investigations: review of blood chemistry.

Clinical assessment using ABCDE

A: Airway

Assess airway and note general impression. Is the woman thirsty? Do her mucous membranes look dry? Does she have a dry mouth, furred tongue, cracked lips? A woman with fluid overload may have wheezing or excessive secretions.

B: Breathing

Assess respiratory rate and measure oxygen saturations.

Deep, rapid respirations may indicate a change in acid base balance as the lungs attempt to 'blow off' extra carbon dioxide. Electrolyte imbalance may cause weakness of respiratory muscles. Crackles, wheezing and/or pink frothy sputum and deteriorating oxygen saturations may indicate pulmonary oedema.

C: Circulation

Measure the vital signs: pulse, blood pressure and temperature.

With fluid depletion, signs of compensatory mechanisms become evident: heart rate increases and, as fluid depletion continues, the blood pressure will drop, although this will be a late sign in a pregnant woman. The woman may complain of feeling dizzy and light-headed (lower the bed flat). The pulse should be taken manually to detect whether it is strong and easily palpable and at a normal rate (healthy) or weak, thready and rapid (volume depletion). Electrolyte imbalance can lead to heart arrhythmias and ECG monitoring will provide further assessment of cardiac function.[6]

Cool skin of hands and feet may indicate peripheral vasoconstriction as the sympathetic nervous system reduces vessel diameter to maintain blood pressure and divert blood to essential organs. Capillary refill time (see Chapter 2) should be less than 2 seconds normally, but will be extended in women with volume depletion. Central venous pressure monitoring may be required.

Hourly urine output measurements are recommended in any unwell woman as they provide a useful assessment of fluid homeostasis. A healthy urine output is around 1 ml/kg/hour, so an average pregnant woman of around 70 kg should produce about 70 ml in an hour. The midwife will also note the degree of concentration of the urine by visual inspection and may also dipstick the urine for assessment of specific gravity. Regular assessment of urine using specimens taken from catheter ports or mid-stream urine samples should be made. A list of information that can be gathered from urine dipstick assessment can be found in Table 3.3. Useful laboratory tests will include

Table 3.3 Information from urine dipstick test[8,9,10]

Specific gravity: normal range 1.016–1.022	Specific gravity estimates the level of solute in the urine and thus reflects the concentration of urine; in volume depletion, the urine would be more concentrated and the reading would be high – for example, 1.030.[8]
pH: usual range 5.5–6.5 but can be normal (4–8)	Not as important as blood pH. Urine infections associated with alkaline urine and abnormalities arise in some renal conditions.
Abnormal constituents	
Blood: may be visible (macroscopic haematuria) or microscopic	Contamination by lochia or blood loss Urethral trauma Kidney or urinary tract disease, calculi, glomerular nephritis Obstructed labour
Protein	Contaminated sample (collect another sample), PET, renal disease, infection, during febrile illness or vigorous exercise
Bilirubin and urobilinogen	Liver or gall bladder disease Abnormal breakdown of red blood cells
Nitrite	Indicates urinary tract infection
Leukocyte esterase (white blood cells)	Pus in urine (mostly neutrophils) indicates urinary tract infection
Glucose	Will appear in urine when blood glucose level above 10 mmol/l approximately; suggests diabetes
Ketones	Suggests excessive fat breakdown; low levels may be normal in pregnancy but are considered an abnormal finding especially in context of fasting, dehydration and uncontrolled diabetes (ketoacidosis)

microscopy, culture and sensitivity (MC&S) (infection) and protein:creatinine ratio (PCR) (pre-eclampsia).

D: Disability

Manifestations of hypovolaemic shock and electrolyte imbalance will affect neurological function. Dizziness and anxiety may occur. Reflexes may be affected. Rising urea can affect level of consciousness.

E: Exposure

Further examination will assess oedema, skin turgor, acute weight changes and blood loss. To assess for oedema, gently press over a bony area for a few seconds and then release. If the indentation created remains for more than 30 seconds, this is called 'pitting' oedema. When assessing pregnant women for oedema, questions should be asked about tightness of rings, changes to facial appearance and history of rapid recent weight gain.

The elasticity of the skin can be assessed by gently pinching an area of skin over a body area such as the back of the hand. If the skin remains raised and does not quickly return to normal, this can indicate fluid depletion.

Investigations

Blood tests that will aid assessment of fluid and electrolyte balance might include:

- Full blood count (FBC): useful to assess for anaemia, sufficient platelets and any indications of infection.
- Blood biochemistry tests (U&Es): urea and creatinine are the two main electrolytes that indicate renal function. The correct levels of sodium and potassium are important for cell function.
- An arterial blood gas may be indicated. This will measure the pH of the blood. A metabolic acidosis is consistent with renal failure (see Chapter 7).

Other tests include chest X-ray and ECG.

Electrolyte imbalance

Sodium, potassium, calcium and magnesium are required for cells to function. If an imbalance of electrolytes occurs, it can give rise to significant cardiac, renal and neuromuscular function. Contraction of heart muscle is dependent on the movement of sodium and potassium through the intracellular to extracellular spaces of heart and nerve cells. The rate of movement is determined by calcium and therefore any disruption to levels of sodium, potassium or calcium have the potential to cause arrhythmias. Hyperkalaemia (high potassium) is the most dangerous.[11] Excess hydrogens (from metabolic acidosis) also depress myocardial contractility. Women will need ECG monitoring and the imbalance will need to be corrected. In PET, reduced systemic arterial pressure in the renal system can lead to sodium and water retention in the kidney. Other signs of electrolyte imbalance include lethargy, muscle weakness, paraesthesia, gastrointestinal symptoms and hypotension.

Fluid replacement

IV fluid administration will improve the volume of fluid within the intravascular compartment (blood vessels), and this in turn has an impact on fluid in the extravascular compartment (interstitial space and cells). Most cases of rapid fluid replacement are given in response to haemorrhage. Fluid overload in cases of pre-eclampsia can lead to life-threatening pulmonary oedema, and fluid restriction with strict hourly input limits need to be observed. This can be challenging when the woman with PET also has substantial blood loss, and in these cases specialised monitoring with CVP may be indicated (see Chapter 2). Women with cardiac conditions and those with sepsis also need particular caution with regard to fluid replacement.

Intravenous access

Short wide-bore (16-gauge) cannulae deliver the fastest flow. They should be inserted into a large peripheral vein, preferably where the cannula doesn't have to transverse a joint. Midwives should insert two wide-bore cannulae as soon as problems arise, and while waiting for medical assistance. Peripheral shutdown will increase as ill health progresses, making it increasingly difficult to gain IV access.

Delivery of infusion

The rate of infusion is usually controlled by the use of volumetric pumps. However, sometimes fluid needs to be replaced quickly and pressure bags are used. This needs to be done with caution, as damage to the vein and surrounding tissue may occur. The midwife should assess the cannula site for any pain, redness or swelling. There is also a risk of delivering too much fluid, too rapidly, causing circulatory overload.[12] Intravenous fluids should be warmed prior to administration as cold fluids will reduce maternal temperature. This will cause shivering and increase metabolic and oxygen demand. Low temperature will cause further peripheral vasoconstriction, which will limit delivery of oxygen to tissues, increasing the risk of acidosis. A reduced temperature also affects the efficiency of coagulation mechanisms [12]

Ongoing assessment to determine the effectiveness of fluid administration.

Regular observations of up to five-minute intervals are indicated when treating shock. Automatic BP monitoring and pulse oximetry will record BP, pulse and saturations. Respiratory rate, temperature and hourly urine output are also indicated. Increased urine output and return of vital signs to normal ranges will indicate improvement. However, if the woman's vital signs do not improve as a result of fluid replacement, there can be a number of reasons that require urgent assessment. The fluid may be moving out of the intravascular compartment and moving into the interstitial space, predisposing the woman to pulmonary oedema. There may be continued loss (as in continued haemorrhage), and further efforts to identify the source of bleeding and take measures to control bleeding, such as bi-manual compression, medication and surgery, are required. There may be increased vasodilation due to worsening sepsis or anaphylaxis, which require specialist vasoactive medication.[12] Critical care specialist involvement is essential. See Box 3.2 for a list of useful assessments and investigations to guide fluid replacement.

Box 3.2 Useful assessments and investigations to guide fluid replacement

- Frequent assessment of vital signs: pulse, respiratory rate, BP, temperature and oxygen saturations;
- Hourly urine output;
- Review of fluid balance;
- Capillary refill;
- Arterial blood gases;
- Assessment of central venous pressure (CVP);
- Advanced monitoring techniques (see Chapter 2).

Types of fluids

There is debate over which is better for fluid replacement: colloids or crystalloids. Both have their place and will be determined by the clinical indication for fluid replacement. They vary in their passage across the capillary structure, which alters the extent and duration of the effect of the infusion. Blood transfusion is often required in cases of significant haemorrhage to replace vital oxygen-carrying red cells.

Crystalloids

Normal saline 0.9%, Hartmann's solution and PlasmaLyte are examples of crystalloid solutions. They contain sodium concentrations similar to those of the extracellular fluid. When given intravenously, they add to the circulating blood volume but their effect is quite short-lived in keeping blood pressure up as they quickly distribute to the interstitial space and cells. There is a risk of fluid overload when administering these fluids in large amounts.

Colloids

Colloids such as Gelofusine and Haemoccel contain large particles. They are effective in increasing blood pressure without needing large volumes of fluid. They achieve this by adding volume to the vascular compartment directly, but they also increase the colloid osmotic pressure in the capillaries, which pulls water from the interstitial compartment, further increasing circulating volume.[8] They are valuable to restore blood volume in cases of significant blood loss, although actual blood replacement is often used as well and therefore they are considered a temporary measure while blood transfusion is arranged. Their benefit in the intravascular compartment lasts for about 1.5 hours.[13] However, there is some controversy regarding their use. They carry a risk of allergic reaction, renal damage and coagulation problems and their use is therefore limited.[12]

Fluid administration in special circumstances

- Haemorrhage
- Pre-eclampsia
- Sepsis
- Cardiac conditions.

Haemorrhage

Blood loss can be rapid in haemorrhage linked to childbirth (see Chapter 5). Box 3.3 gives an example of a suggested fluid regimen. Hospitals should develop clear protocols for management of major obstetric haemorrhage and staff should undertake regular skills drill training.

Box 3.3 Fluid/blood product transfusion guidelines according to RCOG guidelines[14]

- Crystalloid: up to 2 l isotonic crystalloid;

- Colloid: up to 1.5 l colloid until blood arrives;

- Blood: if necessary give group O, RhD-negative, K-negative red cell units (usually routinely kept on delivery suites for emergencies), and change to group-specific red cells as soon as available;

- FFP (fresh frozen plasma): given according to haemostatic testing (or 4 units FFP after 4 units of RBC) if haemorrhage is continuing;

- Platelet concentrations: 1 pool of platelets if platelet count $< 75 \times 10^9$/l and haemorrhage is continuing;

- Cryoprecipitate: 2 pools if fibrinogen < 2 g/l and haemorrhage is continuing.

Pre-eclampsia

Pre-eclampsia poses a particular challenge to fluid balance. It is associated with fluid shift into the interstitial compartment and this is known to predispose to the development of pulmonary oedema. Vasoconstriction secondary to endothelium damage to blood vessels results in – among other symptoms – reduced glomerular filtration, which impacts urine output. The damage to the glomerular capillary membrane within the Bowman's capsule results in loss of protein in the urine, which affects important blood levels of protein that are key in colloid osmotic pressure. Low blood albumin, reduced urine output, increased metabolic wastes in the blood such as raised urates/creatinine, raised blood pressure, increased sensitivity to angiotensin and widespread oedema may all be features of pre-eclampsia.

A major concern is to avoid fluid overload, and most protocols limit input to around 80 ml/hour. If a Syntocinon infusion is required, a concentrated solution delivered via a syringe driver is used. The volume of this and any other infusion (magnesium sulphate, antihypertensives) should be included in the 80 ml/hour total fluids.[15] Drugs used in the management of PET, such as hydralazine and nifedipine, are vasodilators and thus will affect the requirements for circulating volume. Care should be taken with fluids by using low volume bags, and administration via a volumetric pump is recommended.[12] Strict fluid balance records need to be kept, including regular assessment of fluid restrictions and review of hourly urine output. Use of detailed high-dependency charts enable fluid records to be kept alongside records of vital signs. CVP monitoring can be helpful to manage fluid replacement.

Following delivery, symptoms may persist and close monitoring is still required for at least 24 hours. Physiological diuresis will be expected post-delivery and usually indicates recovery.

Sepsis

Hypovolaemia is almost always a feature of sepsis and therefore fluid replacement is essential. The pathophysiology of sepsis means that a large amount of fluid leaks into the interstitial tissues. CVP monitoring may be required to guide fluid replacement

When a woman does not respond to fluid resuscitation, she will require critical care management with vasopressor therapy and ventilation.[12]

Cardiac disease

Great care needs to be taken regarding fluid management for women with cardiac conditions. CVP monitoring or more advanced assessment of cardiac function may be required to guide safe fluid administration.[12]

Blood transfusion

Successful blood transfusion requires careful preparation and checks to ensure safety. During a transfusion, the woman should be cared for where she can be observed and an increased frequency of observations is required to detect any transfusion reaction or complications. Transfusion of packed red blood cells is the most common transfusion given. Table 3.4 gives a summary of the various components of blood that may be given. Table 3.5 gives a summary of blood compatibility. In addition to ABO compatibility, women who are rhesus negative should receive rhesus negative blood, although those who are rhesus positive can receive either rhesus negative or rhesus positive blood.

Informed consent to blood transfusion is required where possible, and the discussion of benefits and risks with the woman documented. The use of blood products requires a clear audit trail whereby components are traceable from donor to final destination.[16]

The biggest risk is receiving the incorrect blood component. There needs to be strict adherence to correct sampling, labelling, cross match and administrative procedures

Table 3.4 Blood components and their administration[9,17]

lood component	Description	Indication	Storage and administration
Red cells	Plasma, white cells and platelets removed, leaving the red cells that contain the haemoglobin	Aims to increase oxygen-carrying capacity by increasing haemoglobin	Stored at 2–6 °C Shelf life 35 days from donation Once collected from blood storage, should be given within 4 hours Usually transfuse over 2–3 hours
Fresh frozen plasma FFP	Coagulation factors	Coagulation factor deficient Major haemorrhage DIC	Stored frozen at −40 °C for up to 12 months When required, is rapidly thawed at 37 °C before issue Once thawed, needs to be transfused within 4 hours, although usually within 30 minutes, as coagulation factors reduce once thawed
Cryoprecipitate	Plasma product rich in clotting factors	To enhance fibrinogen levels in cases of massive haemorrhage and DIC	Stored at −30 °C for up to two years. Once thawed, should be transfused immediately
Platelets	Four donations of platelets are pooled to produce 1 adult unit of platelets	For prevention of haemorrhage in women with low platelet count or platelet dysfunction	Stored on a special agitator rack at 20–4 °C to prevent clumping; expires five days after donation Should not be placed in refrigerator Donor and recipient must be ABO-identical

Table 3.5 Red cell compatibility

Blood group	Red cell antigens	Plasma antibodies	Donor group compatibility
A	A	Anti-B	A and O
B	B	Anti-A	B and O
AB	A and B	None	A, B, AB and O
O	None	Anti-A and anti-B	O

even in an emergency. Wrist bands should contain surname, first name, date of birth and unique identity number. Critical points for checking the identity of the woman are both at the stage of blood sampling and at the point of administration of the blood component. Samples should be labelled at the bedside from wristband details that have been verbally confirmed by the woman.[16,18] See Box 3.4 for details of recommended checks that should be made.

Box 3.4 Checking process of a woman's identity and blood component checks[18,19]

Checks of woman's identity

- Ask the woman to state her full name (first and last names) and date of birth (DOB).
- Check verbal response (full name and DOB) is the same as on the ID band, including spelling.
- Check details on the ID band (full name, DOB and unique identity number) are the same on the hospital notes, prescription chart and request form.
- Check details on the hospital notes and prescription chart (full name, DOB and unique identity number) are the same as on the label attached to the blood unit.

Blood component checks

- Check unique component donation number on the blood unit is the same as on the label attached to blood unit.
- Check blood group on the blood unit is the same as on the label.
- Check the expiry date of the blood component pack label.

Equipment

Adequate IV access using a large-bore 16-gauge needle is generally advised. Blood components should be administered using a specialised blood administration giving set that has an integral filter. It is recommended that the lines are changed at least every 12 hours and at the end of the prescribed transfusion to prevent bacterial growth. A new line is required to transfuse platelets. Rapid infusion of red cells soon after removal from storage (4 °C) can result in hypothermia, and it is therefore advised to use a blood-warming device.[9]

Assessment of a woman receiving a blood transfusion

The woman should be observed directly, with regular assessment, for the duration of a blood transfusion, to enable quick recognition of any adverse transfusion reactions. Most transfusion reactions occur within 30 minutes of starting the transfusion,[18] so close observation during this time is required. Temperature, pulse, blood pressure and respiratory rate should be recorded within 15 minutes of the transfusion beginning – earlier if a rapid transfusion. Prior to the infusion (within 60 minutes of the infusion), a set of baseline observations of temperature, pulse, blood pressure and respiratory rate should be recorded.[16] This serves two purposes: first, to act as a comparison to monitor the effectiveness of the transfusion, and second, to identify subsequent changes that would indicate a transfusion reaction. A further set of observations should be recorded following the transfusion and any routine observations then continued.[16]

Transfusion reactions

There are three main types of complications and reactions to blood transfusion:

- Receiving the wrong blood or an incompatible transfusion;
- Having an allergic or anaphylactic reaction to the blood;
- Receiving blood that is contaminated with either a bacterial or viral infection.

Acute transfusion reactions can vary from mild febrile reactions to life-threatening allergic, haemolytic or hypotensive events.[20] Types of transfusion reactions and symptoms are listed in Table 3.6.

Acute transfusion reactions may begin immediately after the transfusion starts. In all cases, the immediate management is to stop the infusion, undertake an ABCDE assessment and respond accordingly. If severe, call for urgent medical help. Transfer to a higher-level care facility will be required. The details of the transfused unit should be checked against the woman's details to ascertain if the right blood has been given to the correct woman. Seek advice from the medical practitioner and alert haematology. Return blood components, including the giving set, to the blood transfusion department.[20] More frequent observations, including oxygen saturations and urine output, should be made to monitor maternal wellbeing.

Table 3.6 Types of transfusion reactions[9,17,20,21]

Type of reaction	Signs and symptoms	Response
Acute transfusion reaction	Fever	Stop the transfusion.
	Chills	These can be mild, moderate or severe.
	Rigors	Assess ABCDE and respond accordingly –
	Tachycardia	if severe, call for urgent medical help, as may lead to life-threatening acute renal failure and DIC.
	Hyper/hypotension	
	Collapse	
	Flushing	Seek advice from haematologist.
	Urticaria	Check ID/blood compatibility label.
	Pain (loin, bone, muscle, chest, abdomen)	Look for turbidity, clots, discolouration.
	Respiratory distress, nausea, general malaise	Monitor closely; may require admission to higher-level care facility.

continued

Table 3.6 continued

Type of reaction	Signs and symptoms	Response
		If mild: isolated temperature and rash only – may continue transfusion after advice sought and increase observations.
		Causes such as wrong blood, anaphylaxis and bacterial contamination are to be considered.
Infusion of bacterial contaminated unit	Rigors Pyrexia Hypo/hypertension Tachycardia Collapse	Stop the transfusion ABCDE assessment and response. Take blood cultures. Contact microbiologist and administer IV antibiotics. Alert Haematology.
Transfusion-related acute lung injury (TRALI) Symptoms usually occur within 6 hours	Acute breathlessness Non-productive cough Hypotension Low white cells count Chest X-ray shows features similar to acute respiratory chest syndrome	Stop the transfusion ABCDE assessment and response. It may be difficult to distinguish from alternative diagnoses such as cardiac conditions or pulmonary oedema. Treatment will include oxygen and mechanical ventilation may be required.
Transfusion-associated circulatory overload (TACO)	Any four of the following occurring within 6 hours of transfusion: acute respiratory distress; tachycardia; hypertension; pulmonary oedema; evidence of positive fluid balance	Stop the transfusion if still in progress and stop any IV fluids. ABCDE assessment and response. Manage as for circulatory overload. Place woman in upright position and give oxygen. Keep monitoring fluid balance and fluid restriction.
Allergic reactions or anaphylaxis Usually symptoms occur at start of transfusion	Hypotension Bronchospasm Chest or abdominal pain Difficulty breathing Nausea/vomiting Urticaria Flushed appearance, redness of skin Swelling around eyes Laryngeal oedema	Stop the transfusion ABCDE assessment and response. Administration of IM adrenaline according to Resuscitation Guidelines UK.[22]
Post-transfusion purpura	Bruising and bleeding 5–12 days after transfusion Low platelet count	Caused by platelet-specific alloantibodies. Treatment immunoglobulin.

Further reading

British Committee for Standards in Haematology (BSH). 2009. Guideline on the administration of blood components. Available at www.b-s-h.org.uk/media/15782/admin_blood_components-bcsh-05012010.pdf. Accessed 10 September 2017. (Detailed evidence-based guidance on administration of blood products.)

Tinegate, H, Birchall, J, Gray, A, Haggas, R, Massey, E, Norfolk, D . . . and Allard, S. 2012. Guideline on the investigation and management of acute transfusion reactions. *British Journal of Haematology*, *159*(2): 143–53. (Guidance for the recognition and management of acute transfusion reactions. Has useful flow diagram to distinguish management between mild, moderate and severe reactions.)

Watson, D and Hearnshaw, K. 2010. Understanding blood groups and transfusion in nursing practice. *Nursing Standard*, *24*(30): 41–8. (Easy-to-read summary of keys areas of blood transfusion.)

References

1. McGloin, S. 2015. The ins and outs of fluid balance in the acutely ill patient. *British Journal of Nursing*, *24*(1): 14–18.
2. Lewis, G (ed.). 2007. The confidential enquiry into maternal and child health (CEMACH). Saving mothers' lives: reviewing maternal deaths to make motherhood safer – 2003–2005. The seventh report on confidential enquiries into maternal deaths in the United Kingdom. London: CEMACH.
3. Centre for Maternal and Child Enquiries (CMACE). 2011. Saving mothers' lives: reviewing maternal deaths to make motherhood safer: 2006–2008. The eighth report on confidential enquiries into maternal deaths in the United Kingdom. *British Journal of Obstetrics and Gynaecology*, *118*(1): s1–203.
4. Harding, K, Redmond, P and Tuffnell, D on behalf of the MBRRACE-UK hypertensive disorders of pregnancy chapter writing group. 2016. Caring for women with hypertensive disorders of pregnancy. In: Knight, M, Nour, M, Tuffnell, D, Kenyon, S, Shakespeare, J, Brocklehurst, P and Kurinczuk, JJ (eds) on behalf of MBRRACE-UK. *Saving lives, improving mothers' care: surveillance of maternal deaths in the UK 2012–14 and lessons learned to inform maternity care from the UK and Ireland confidential enquiries into maternal deaths and morbidity 2009–14*. Oxford, UK: National Perinatal Epidemiology Unit, University of Oxford, pp. 69–75.
5. Scales, K and Pilsworth, J. 2008. The importance of fluid balance in clinical practice. *Nursing Standard*, *22*(47): 50–7.
6. Allibone, L. 2012. Body fluids and electrolytes. In: Peate, I and Dutton, H (eds). *Recognising and responding to medical emergencies*. Harlow, UK: Pearson, pp. 59 80.
7. Rowe, N. 2007. Fluid balance and management and the critically ill woman. In: Billington, M and Stevenson, M (eds). *Critical care in childbearing for midwives*. Oxford, UK: Blackwell Publishing, pp. 167–77.
8. Finch, J. 2012. The patient with acute renal problems. In: Peate, I and Dutton, H (eds). *Recognising and responding to medical emergencies*. Harlow, UK: Pearson, pp. 183–205.
9. Jevon, P and Ewens, B. 2012. *Monitoring the critically ill patient*. Oxford, UK: Wiley-Blackwell.
10. Higgins, C. 2013. *Understanding laboratory investigations: a guide for nurses, midwives and healthcare professionals*. Oxford, UK: Wiley-Blackwell.
11. Donald, R. 2011. Caring for the renal system. In: Macintosh, M and Moore, T (eds). *Caring for the seriously ill patient*. London: Hodder Arnold.
12. Paterson-Brown, S and Howell, C (eds). 2016. *The MOET course manual: managing obstetric emergencies and trauma*. Cambridge, UK: Cambridge University Press.

13. Vaughan, D, Robinson, N, Lucas, N and Arulkumaran, S. 2010. *Handbook of obstetric high dependency care*. Chichester, UK: Blackwell Publishing.
14. Mavrides, E, Allard, S, Chandraharan, E, Collins, P, Green, L, Hunt, BJ . . . and Thomson, AJ on behalf of the Royal College of Obstetricians and Gynaecologists. 2016. Prevention and management of postpartum haemorrhage. *British Journal of Obstetrics and Gynaecology, 124*: 106–49.
15. National Institute for Health and Care Excellence (NICE). 2010. Hypertension in pregnancy: diagnosis and management. Available at www.nice.org.uk/guidance/cg107/resources/hypertension-in-pregnancy-diagnosis-and-management-pdf-35109334009285. Accessed 24 September 2017.
16. British Committee for Standards in Haematology (BSH). 2009. Guideline on the administration of blood components. Available at www.b-s-h.org.uk/media/15782/admin_blood_components-bcsh-05012010.pdf. Accessed 10 September 2017.
17. Watson, D and Hearnshaw, K. 2010. Understanding blood groups and transfusion in nursing practice. *Nursing Standard, 24*(30): 41–8.
18. Bolton-Maggs, PHB (ed.) on behalf of the Serious Hazards of Transfusion (SHOT) Steering Group. 2017. The 2016 annual SHOT report. Available at www.shotuk.org/wp-content/uploads/SHOT-Report-2016_web_11th-July.pdf. Accessed 20 March 2018.
19. Swann, T. 2010. Royal Berkshire NHS Trust: trust policy for blood transfusion. Available at www.transfusionguidelines.org/document.../rtc-scent_policy_tx_berks.pdf. Accessed 10 September 2017.
20. Tinegate, H, Birchall, J, Gray, A, Haggas, R, Massey, E, Norfolk, D . . . and Allard, S. 2012. Guideline on the investigation and management of acute transfusion reactions. *British Journal of Haematology, 159*(2): 143–53.
21. Watson, D and Denison, C. 2014. Recognising and managing transfusion reactions. *Nursing Times, 110*(39): 18–21.
22. Resuscitation Council (UK) Emergency treatment of anaphylactic reactions: guidelines for healthcare providers. Available at www.resus.org.uk/anaphylaxis/emergency-treatment-of-anaphylactic-reactions/ accessed. 10 September 2017.

Chapter 4

Shock

Introduction

Shock is defined as the inability of the circulation to deliver essential oxygen and nutrients to the cells. Insufficient oxygen results in life-threatening cellular dysfunction. Box 4.1 lists causes of shock in pregnant and postpartum women.

Box 4.1 Causes of shock in pregnant and postpartum women[1,2]

- Postural hypotension: obstruction of blood flow as a result of the gravid uterus impeding on major blood vessels. Women in later stages of pregnancy should lie in lateral position or be tilted 30°.
- Hypotension due to the vasodilating effects of regional anaesthesia.
- Hypovolaemic: decreased circulating blood volume as a result of haemorrhage such as PPH (see Chapter 5).
- Cardiogenic: impaired cardiac function, such as myocardial infarction, cardiomyopathy or arrhythmias (see Chapter 8).
- Septic shock: dysregulation of the immune response to infection.
- Anaphylaxis: inflammatory response subsequent to hypersensitivity to an allergen (allergic response).
- Amniotic fluid embolism: not strictly classified as shock but included here as features similar to anaphylaxis.
- Neurogenic: vasodilation associated with autonomic nervous system dysfunction or sedation following anaesthesia, causing depression of respiratory centre or circulatory system (see Chapter 9).
- Pulmonary embolism: obstructive shock caused by reduction in venous return to the heart and reduced oxygenation (see Chapter 7).

Hypovolaemic shock subsequent to antepartum or postpartum haemorrhage is the most common form of shock that midwives will encounter. The details of assessment in relation to haemorrhage are included in a dedicated chapter on this subject (see Chapter 5). The 'Confidential enquiry into maternal deaths' report[3] indicated high rates of morbidity and mortality attributed to cardiac conditions in pregnancy. Recognition and assessment of undiagnosed and known cardiac conditions, some of which will lead to cardiogenic shock, are also discussed in a separate chapter (see Chapter 8).

Sepsis or septic shock has always posed a risk to pregnant and postpartum women, and a recent increase in cases has prompted the development of a new set of assessment tools to aid early recognition and prompt referral.[4,5] The majority of this chapter will review assessment to prevent and treat life-threatening maternal sepsis. The recognition of rarer causes of shock/collapse – anaphylaxis and amniotic fluid embolism – are also included.

Pathophysiology of shock

In cases of shock, the woman's body will attempt to compensate by initiating the sympathetic nervous system fight or flight response. This reaction aims to maintain oxygen supply to vital organs such as the brain and heart. In physiological terms, the uterus, and consequently the fetus, is not considered a vital organ, and blood is diverted away from the placenta. Fetal distress is therefore a sensitive and early sign of maternal deteriorating health. Table 4.1 describes the stages of shock from the body's initial recognition that there is a problem through compensatory mechanisms to maintain homeostasis, with the progressive and refractory stages signifying an immediate life-threatening state. There is a window of opportunity for the midwife to recognise

Table 4.1 Stages of shock

Stages of shock	Features
Initial	Fall in blood pressure will be identified by pressure sensors in aorta and carotid arteries.
	Autonomic nervous system responds by signalling peripheral blood vessels to constrict, which will increase blood volume in central circulation and oxygen will be delivered to vital areas such as heart, brain and muscles; a woman may be noted to appear pale but will otherwise feel well.
	Fetal tachycardia or other signs of fetal distress can be an early sign of maternal shock.
Compensatory	Release of adrenaline and noradrenaline (fight or flight) response will now result in increased pulse rate, cold peripheries and nausea as blood is diverted from non-vital areas of skin and GIT; the respiratory rate will increase in response to build-up of lactic acid; this compensatory respiratory alkalosis may result in an altered mental state such as confusion or aggression; there will be reduced urine output as the kidneys respond to preserve fluid.
Progressive	Compensatory mechanisms start to fail.
	Tissue ischaemia and hypoxia.
	Shock is still reversible in early stages, but intensive intervention required.
Refractory	Cell death, tissue death, multiple organ dysfunction and death inevitable

characteristic signs and symptoms of the compensatory stage. This allows timely intervention to avoid more serious illness.

In untreated shock, the cells will react to a lack of oxygen by producing the required energy, adenosine triphosphate (ATP), by anaerobic means. This is inefficient and produces lactic acid. A build-up of lactic acid causes a metabolic acidosis, and the body responds to this by increasing the respiratory rate to try to 'blow off' the excess carbon dioxide. Pregnant and postnatal women, due to their age, general health and fluid excess, are known to compensate well. While this is good, it creates a problem in that there can be a delay in detecting critical ill health, and, by the time they display symptoms, their condition is serious. Table 4.2 gives a summary of the symptoms associated with various types of shock more commonly seen in maternity settings.

Table 4.2 Clinical features found on assessment of various types of shock[1,2]

Assessment	Hypovolaemia	Sepsis	Cardiogenic	Anaphylaxis	Neurogenic
Skin colour and appearance	Pale Cool skin Sweaty Delayed capillary refill	Initially flushed with warm skin (profound vasodilation), later pale and cool extremities Features of infection	Grey/ cyanosed Cold and clammy skin	Redness, flushing Swelling to face and neck Blistering wheals/pruritus Warm skin Nausea, diarrhoea, vomiting Onset usually within minutes of exposure to allergen	Pale Warm skin
Behaviour and level of consciousness	Restless, agitated Anxious Thirsty	Confusion	Drowsy, confused Chest pain	Altered LOC Extreme anxiety or panic Collapse	Altered LOC
Respiratory symptoms	Tachypnoea	Tachypnoea	Tachypnoea Shortness of breath Orthopnoea Basal pulmonary crackles	Tachypnoea Stridor due to laryngeal oedema Wheeze due to bronchospasm	Bradypnoea
Pulse	Tachycardia	Tachycardia	Tachycardia	Tachycardia	Bradycardia
Blood pressure	Hypotension (late sign)	Hypotension	Hypotension	Hypotension	Hypotension
Urine output	Reduced urine output	Reduced urine output	Reduced urine output	Reduced urine output	Reduced urine output
Central venous pressure	Reduced CVP	Reduced CVP	Elevated CVP Raised jugular venous pressure	Reduced CVP	
ECG			Cardiac arrhythmias		

Sepsis

Reports arising from the 'Confidential enquiry into maternal deaths'[6,7,8] have noted a significant increase in maternal mortality and morbidity due to sepsis. They have emphasised the need for awareness of the symptoms of sepsis, early recognition and prompt referral of women, with a 'back-to-basics' approach advocated that includes acknowledgement of risk factors, careful clinical assessment and recording of vital signs.

Sepsis is defined as 'life-threatening organ dysfunction caused by a dysregulated host response to infection'.[9] Something to note in this definition is, first, that sepsis is life-threatening and therefore requires urgent referral by the midwife for medical review and action. Second, the features of sepsis arise from an inappropriate control of the woman's normal responses to inflammation. These 'red flag' features need to be identified by the midwife by ensuring a full assessment of the woman is carried out. Third, sepsis arises from a source infection and that source will need to be identified and treated.[10]

Septic shock is a progression of sepsis where there is significant and persistent reduction in blood pressure and abnormalities of cell function.[9]

Pathophysiology of the development of sepsis

In sepsis, the normal response to infection of vasodilation, leaky capillaries and clot formation are exaggerated.[2] In the presence of invading pathogenic bacteria, the immune system activates macrophages and neutrophils as well as other factors such as cytokines, tumour necrosis factor and interleukins. This is usually effective at controlling the spread of infection. In situations where there are lots of bacteria or the regulatory response is out of control, inflammation becomes generalised, resulting in severe sepsis. The inflammatory mediators act on the endothelial lining of blood vessels, causing increased capillary permeability and an increased production of the powerful vasodilator, nitric acid. The blood vessels dilate and fluid moves into the interstitial space, causing a significant drop in blood pressure. Anaerobic metabolism due to oxygen deficiency in the cells starts to produce lactic acid. Compensatory mechanisms, such as an increased heart rate and an increased respiratory rate, aim to increase cardiac output and correct acidosis, but as these compensatory mechanisms fail to work, underperfusion to the organs occurs and organs such as the kidneys and heart start to fail. The fluid shift caused by sepsis puts the woman at risk of pulmonary oedema. In sepsis, there will be reduced blood flow to the uterus, with consequent reduced oxygenation to the fetus, and signs of fetal distress or demise may be evident.

A second wave of cytokine responses in sepsis involves the release of platelets and stimulation of the coagulation, complement and kinin systems. Platelet aggregation is triggered by endothelial damage. This activation of the coagulation system can result in disseminated intravascular coagulation (DIC). The tendency towards clot formation, on top of already-existing pro-coagulation of pregnancy, predisposes pregnant and postpartum women with sepsis to microvascular clot formation. The combination of ischaemia from low blood pressure and clot formation will result in further organ dysfunction.

Clinical features of sepsis

Signs and symptoms

There are two phases recognised in the progress of septic shock: warm shock (initial vasodilation) followed by cold shock (as compensatory mechanisms start to fail). Box 4.2 lists the features of the progressive stages of septic shock and organ dysfunction.

Box 4.2 Features of septic shock and organ dysfunction[11]

Initial: warm shock
- Warm peripheries (peripheral vasodilation);
- Low blood pressure;
- Raised and bounding heart rate;
- Temperature instability;
- Increased respiratory rate;
- Altered mental state.

Late stages: cold shock
- Cold peripheries (peripheral vasoconstriction);
- Sweating;
- Weak, thready pulse.

Organ dysfunction
- Impaired renal function: oliguria, electrolyte imbalance, raised creatinine;
- Neurological compromise: confusion, agitation and possibly coma;
- Cardiopulmonary impairment: cyanosis and adult respiratory distress syndrome;
- Haematological changes: reduced platelet count, disseminated intravascular coagulation;
- Metabolic acidosis with raised serum lactate;
- Liver impairment: increased serum bilirubin and increased alkaline phosphatase;
- Gastrointestinal: diarrhoea, paralytic ileus.

Risk factors for developing sepsis

Pregnant and postpartum women are vulnerable to developing sepsis. Interventions in labour, relative immune suppression of pregnancy, enhanced blood supply to the uterus, surgery, wounds and urinary catheterisation are a few reasons why childbirth increases the risk of sepsis. Pre-existing medical conditions such as diabetes, sickle cell disease, HIV and obesity increase vulnerability to infection. See Box 4.3 for a list of risk factors for development of infection and sepsis. However, sepsis can occur in previously-healthy women following uncomplicated pregnancy and vaginal birth.[12] Group A Streptococcus (GAS) has been identified as a particularly virulent infection affecting the genital tract. CMACE[8] highlighted the potential risk of sepsis following contact with young children who had a sore throat or upper respiratory tract infection. Advice was given that women should wash their hands both before and after using the toilet to avoid contamination of the perineal area.

However, causes of maternal sepsis are not limited to infections relating directly to childbirth. In fact, the most common cause of sepsis deaths in pregnant and postpartum women in recent years has been due to influenza[6,7] (see Chapter 7).

Box 4.3 Risk factors for development of infection and sepsis[13,14,15,16]

Features of the women:

- Medical conditions: diabetes, HIV, sickle cell disease, obesity;
- Women from minority and poor socio-economic groups;
- Women for whom language was a barrier to receiving care.

Pregnancy:

- Septic miscarriage or termination of pregnancy;
- Cervical suture;
- Prolonged spontaneous rupture of membranes (especially if preterm);
- Amniocentesis or other invasive procedures.

Labour and puerperium:

- Induction of labour;
- Preterm birth;
- Caesarean section or instrumental vaginal delivery;
- Prolonged rupture of membranes or chorioamnionitis;
- Retained products of conception;
- Urinary tract infection and/or catheterisation;
- Mastitis;
- Close contact with someone with Group A streptococcus – for example, a child with a throat infection.

Assessment of women with regard to sepsis

The identification of sepsis may begin with an initial recognition that the woman is 'not quite right'. Symptoms of sepsis may be less distinctive and may progress more rapidly in pregnant and postpartum women.[17,18] The woman's family may seek help because they feel the woman is displaying unusual behaviour – 'not herself'.

Sepsis is a complex syndrome and some of the symptoms can be vague and overlap with other clinical conditions such as ectopic pregnancy, placental abruption and gastroenteritis. Midwives need to be alert to signs of sepsis by performing a regular

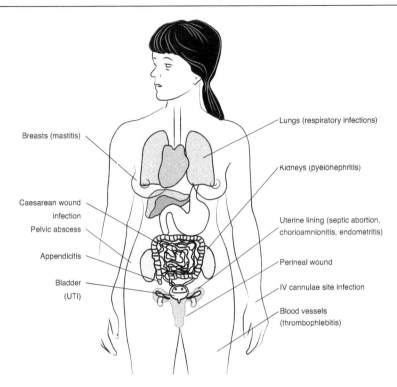

Figure 4.1 Sites of infection that may predispose to sepsis in pregnant and postpartum women

Source: Judy Bothamley and Maureen Boyle. 2015. *Infections affecting pregnancy and childbirth.* Boca Raton, FL: CRC Press.

set of observations, particularly on women who appear unwell and/or have risk factors such as prolonged rupture of membranes, possible incomplete delivery of the placenta, uterine tenderness or sub-involution. Assessment involves a general assessment to identify features of ill health related to the dysregulated immune response; however, it is also important to identify the source of the infection, and this requires a head-to-toe approach. Figure 4.1 indicates potential sites of infection that may predispose to sepsis in pregnant and postpartum women.

Assessment by the midwife will therefore involve:

- identifying risk factors for sepsis by review of the maternity notes or through questioning (Box 4.3);
- structured set of basic observations to determine any physiological features outside of normal parameters, based on ABCD;
- head-to-toe examination (E) to further evaluate wellbeing and identify any existing source of infection.

Basic observations and ABCD assessment

The midwife will start her examination by asking the woman how she feels. The evaluation of the woman's response to this question covers a number of aspects of an Airway,

Breathing, Circulation (ABC) assessment, both in the content of her response and the physical aspects of the way she communicates. She may seem unwell, have some difficulty breathing, be in pain, or have characteristics of an infection with or without a temperature.[5] One of the earliest signs of ill health is an increased respiratory rate. The respiratory rate will go up in response to pyrexia and lactic acidosis, and measurement of oxygen saturations will provide useful information of respiratory and circulatory function.

The midwife will then perform and record a basic set of observations including temperature, pulse, respiratory rate, oxygen saturations and blood pressure. Where the midwife is concerned about the woman, it is helpful that the midwife makes these observations face-to-face. Subtle changes such as a bounding pulse (subsequent to vasodilation, an inflammatory response) or thready pulse (later sign of septic shock as peripheral shutdown occurs to conserve blood pressure) will be felt.[10] When the pulse is taken, what does her skin feel like – cold, hot, clammy, sweaty? (see Table 4.2 for various features of different types of shock.) Does she look pale or flushed? Is there any rash? Can the midwife detect any unusual odours – malodorous lochia, the smell of diarrhoea?[10,13]

An increased temperature is associated with infection, but in sepsis, due to the abnormal immune response and compensatory changes, a normal temperature or hypothermia can be found. When assessing the temperature, the midwife should enquire if the woman has taken any antipyretic medication such as paracetamol.[10] Compensatory mechanisms will mean the woman's blood pressure will not drop until sepsis has progressed into septic shock. Frequent monitoring of BP is indicated using an automated device.

Neurological impairment, such as confusion, may be an early clinical sign that is noted by caregivers and family. AVPU assessment (see Chapter 9) should be included in vital signs observations.

Urine output is a useful indicator of circulation. Where the woman is exhibiting signs of deterioration, insertion of a urinary catheter and hourly urometer should be considered to measure urine output accurately.

In hospital, the midwife may refer to any records of urine output and fluid balance. A sample of urine should be sent for microscopy, culture and sensitivity (MC&S).

The observations should be plotted on a modified early obstetric warning system (MEOWS) chart to enable triggers for ill health to be identified easily and to monitor trends. These charts should not replace, but rather supplement, effective clinical assessment. The Sepsis Trust,[4] in conjunction with NICE,[5] has produced useful checklists with red and amber alerts and algorithms for actions. The 'UK Sepsis Trust community midwifery sepsis screening and action tool' is reproduced here with permission. Note the maternal 'red' and 'amber' features that will prompt action by the midwife to summon an urgent medical review (see Figure 4.2).

Head-to-toe examination (E)

Further assessment will include a review of the clinical history, review of the notes and observation charts and any relevant results from investigations. The midwife will want to know the stage of pregnancy/postnatal, details of the labour, fetal/newborn wellbeing and other features to identify risk factors. In sepsis, the head-to-toe

Community Midwifery Sepsis Screening and Action Tool

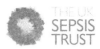

To be applied to all women who are pregnant (or have been pregnant in the last 6 weeks irrespective of outcome) with fever (or recent fever) symptoms or who have unexplained illness

1. In the context of presumed infection, are any of the following true:

(common sources: pneumonia, UTI, breast abscess/ mastitis, endometritis, chorioamnionitis, infected caesarean or perineal wound, influenza, intra-abdominal infection)

	Tick
Patient looks, or says they are, very unwell	☐
Family or carer is very concerned	☐
There is ongoing deterioration	☐

N → Low risk of sepsis. Consider other diagnoses. Use clinical judgement and/or standard protocols.

Give safety netting advice to patient & family; call 999 if deteriorates rapidly, call 111/ arrange to see GP if condition fails to improve or gradually worsens. Signpost to available resources as appropriate. Consider obstetric assessment

↑ N

Y ↓

Perform a full set of observations: NEWS is valid after delivery

3. Is any Maternal Amber Flag present?

	Tick
Relatives worried about mental state/ behaviour	☐
Acute deterioration in functional ability	☐
Respiratory rate 21-24 OR very breathless	☐
Heart rate 91-129 OR new dysrhythmia	☐
Systolic BP 91-100 mmHg	☐
Not passed urine in last 12-18 hours	☐
Temperature < 36°C	☐
Immunosuppressed/ diabetes/ gestational diabetes	☐
Has had invasive procedure in last 6 weeks	☐
(e.g. CS, forceps delivery, ERPC, cerclage, CVs, miscarriage, termination)	
Prolonged rupture of membranes	☐
Close contact with GAS	☐
Bleeding/ offensive wound/ vaginal discharge	☐

If immunity also impaired treat as Red Flag Sepsis

2. Is ONE maternal Red Flag present?

	Tick
Responds only to voice or pain/ unresponsive	☐
Acute confusion	☐
Systolic B.P ≤ 90 mmHg	☐
Heart rate ≥ 130 per minute	☐
Respiratory rate ≥ 25 per minute	☐
Needs oxygen to keep SpO₂ ≥92%	☐
Non-blanching rash, mottled/ ashen/ cyanotic	☐
Not passed urine in last 18 hours	☐

N →

↓ Y

At risk of sepsis

1. Same day assessment by GP/ Team Leader
2. Is urgent hospital referral required?
3. Agree and document ongoing management plan (including observations frequency, planned second review as agreed with GP / Team Leader)
4. Monitor urine output
Consider life threatening sepsis mimics e.g. P.E.

Y ↓

Red Flag Sepsis! This is a time critical condition, immediate action is required.

1. Dial 999, arrange blue light transfer
2. If available give O₂ to keep saturations >94%
3. Cannulate if skills & competencies allow
4. Consider IV fluids
5. Inform family
6. Ensure crew pre-alert as 'Red Flag Sepsis'

Sepsis Six and Red Flag Sepsis are copyright to and intellectual property of the UK Sepsis Trust; registered charity no. 1158843. **sepsistrust.org**

Figure 4.2 UK Sepsis Trust: community midwifery sepsis screening and action tool[4]

Source: Reproduced with permission of the UK Sepsis Trust

Box 4.4 Swabs and specimens that may be useful in investigating the source of infection[18]

Swabs

- Throat
- High vaginal swab
- CS or perineal wound site
- From the neonate

Specimens

- Midstream urine (MSU), catheter specimen urine (CSU)
- Placenta
- Sputum
- Cerebrospinal fluid (CSF) (from a lumbar puncture)
- Expressed breast milk
- Stool sample.

---

examination is important to identify the source of infection. Collecting swabs for microbiological examination can be done at the same time (see Box 4.4). Box 4.5 gives details of some signs of illness and some infections and their features midwives might note during head-to-toe examination. Genital tract sepsis can present as constant severe abdominal or perineal pain and tenderness that is disproportionate to that which would normally be expected, and which is not relieved by usual analgesic medication. Diarrhoea in addition to this pain is characteristic of sepsis.[14,17] In pregnancy, maternal infection will quickly affect the fetus, and an abnormal heart rate pattern may indicate maternal disease.[14]

Group A streptococcus (GAS) is a particularly serious, life-threatening organism that women may acquire from family members, particularly children. Midwives should enquire about possible infection among family members.

Investigations, management and ongoing assessment of sepsis

The 'Surviving sepsis campaign' is an international effort to improve recognition and management of sepsis.[19] Clinicians should refer to the full guidance. In addition, the RCOG have developed guidelines on management of sepsis specific for pregnancy and the puerperium.[17,18] These documents and details of how to access them are listed under 'Further reading' at the end of the chapter. Multidisciplinary management with senior clinical leadership will be needed to direct care. The team, in addition to senior maternity unit staff, will include an intensive care specialist, general surgeon, microbiologist and the critical care outreach team. Admission to intensive care unit (ICU) will be indicated by the woman's condition.

As a memory aid, the management of sepsis is summarised as the 'sepsis six'[20] (see Box 4.6). Investigations will underpin diagnosis and guide treatment (see Box 4.7). Prompt treatment with an adequate dose of appropriate IV antibiotics is essential. The aim is that antibiotics should start within 1 hour of suspecting sepsis and after samples have been obtained for cultures. While awaiting medical aid, the midwife should give oxygen if available to maintain oxygen saturations above 94%, gain

Box 4.5 Head-to-toe assessment to identify features
of infections that may lead to sepsis in pregnant and postpartum
women

Increased temperature, heart rate, pain, muscle aching and general feelings of malaise
and fatigue are features of infection but, depending on the site and causative organism,
other more specific features may be noted:

- Neurological: *meningitis*: characteristic rash, photophobia, headache. Confusion
  is an early feature of sepsis.
- Breasts: *infective mastitis* or *breast abscess*: cracked nipples, reddened wedge-
  shaped discolouration indicating a blocked duct, pain and pus.
- Respiratory: *respiratory infection, pneumonia*: cough, sputum, abnormal breath
  sounds, increased respiratory rate. Acidosis results in increased respiratory rate.
- Uterus: *chorioamnionitis*: malodorous-smelling cloudy amniotic fluid, fetal and
  maternal tachycardia. *Endometritis*: delayed involution of the uterus, malodorous
  and/or heavy lochia, abdominal pain.
- Wounds: normal wound healing involves inflammatory processes of redness,
  swelling, pain and warmth, but, where there is increasing redness, swelling, pain,
  exudate and delayed healing accompanied by systemic features of infection, an
  infection of the wound is likely.
- Abdomen: *pelvic abscess, appendicitis* and *cholecystitis*: unusual level and pattern
  of pain.
- Skin: warm (high temperature), unusual rashes, jaundice and inflammation around
  IV cannula sites. Pale, cold, clammy skin indicative of compensatory shock and
  significant ill health. Areas where the skin or mucosa has been broken, such as
  intravenous cannulae sites, CS or perineal wounds, drains or arterial line sites,
  should be examined and swabs taken of any discharge.
- Urinary tract: malodourous, cloudy urine. Leucocytes and protein may be found
  on dipstick of midstream or catheter specimen of urine. Radiating flank pain may
  be indicative of *pyelonephritis*. Symptoms of urinary infection, such as frequency,
  urgency and pain on passing urine, may not be present in pregnancy. Quantity
  of urine output needs to be assessed.
- Bowels: diarrhoea noted as feature of sepsis.
- Legs: *thrombophlebitis*: pain and swelling.

IV access and consider giving IV fluids. This will be a frightening experience for the
woman and her family and the midwife will need to provide information, support
and clear guidance. Ongoing assessment by the midwife will include frequent
observations of vital signs, including oxygen saturations, neurological assessment,
careful records of administration of fluids to prevent fluid overload, assessment of
fetal wellbeing and general assessment of the woman's response to treatment.

Box 4.6 'Sepsis six'[20]

- Give oxygen to keep saturations above 94%;
- Take blood cultures;
- Give IV antibiotics;
- Give IV fluids and monitor response;
- Measure lactate levels;
- Measure urine output.

Box 4.7 Investigations for sepsis[2,18]

- Blood culture;
- Serum lactate;
- FBC and C-reactive protein (CRP);
- Renal and liver function tests;
- Coagulation screen;
- Samples and swabs taken as indicated by clinical suspicion of the focus of infection;
- Imaging – chest X-ray, pelvic USS, CT scan.

Anaphylaxis

Introduction

Anaphylaxis is a severe, life-threating, systemic hypersensitivity reaction to a substance to which the woman has become sensitised.[21] See Box 4.8 for some of the triggers known to cause anaphylaxis. The reaction causes the rapid release of inflammatory mediators, most significantly mast cells and basophils, which release histamine.[22]

Box 4.8 Triggers for anaphylaxis[21]

- Food: most commonly nuts, but can be milk, seafood, fruit and other foods.
- Drugs: antibiotics, anaesthetic drugs and non-steroidal anti-inflammatory drugs (NSAIDs) are the most common. All drugs have the potential to cause anaphylaxis, and those given IV will cause reactions more rapidly than those ingested.
- Stings/venom: wasp and bee stings most common.
- Other substances: contrast media used in radiology, latex.

Airway and/or breathing and/or circulation problems rapidly develop, typically with accompanying skin and mucosal changes. Fluid shift from the intravascular compartment into the tissues can usually be seen externally as severe tissue swelling (commonly facial), and internally causes laryngeal and pulmonary oedema.[23] Severe upper airway obstruction due to oedema can lead to asphyxiation. Tachycardia, cardiac arrhythmias and reduced cardiac contractility may occur.

It is a rare event. Estimates suggest the incidence of maternal anaphylaxis is approximately 1 in 30,000 pregnancies, although it is thought that the incidence is increasing.[24] Documentation of any allergy must be made clear within the woman's maternity notes and on the prescription chart.

Clinical features

Key features of anaphylaxis are:

* symptoms that are sudden and progress rapidly;
* life-threatening Airway, Breathing and/or Circulation problems;
* skin and/or mucosal changes.

See Table 4.3 for features of anaphylaxis.

Table 4.3 Features of anaphylaxis[21,25]

A Airway	Airway swelling – throat and tongue swelling; feeling as though throat is closing up
	Swelling to lips and face
	Hoarse voice
	Stridor
B Breathing	Shortness of breath
	Wheeze
	Can lead to cyanosis and respiratory arrest
C Circulation	Signs of shock – cold and clammy
	Tachycardia
	Hypotension
	Can have gastrointestinal symptoms – abdominal pain, incontinence, vomiting
	ECG changes, (or CTG may reflect fetal distress)
	Cardiac arrest
D Disability	Confusion, agitation due to hypoxia, decreased level of consciousness
	A preceding 'feeling of impending doom'[26]
E Exposure	Skin and mucosal changes are the first feature in over 80% of anaphylactic reactions; can be subtle or dramatic; range from a generalised red rash to urticaria (inflamed wheals or welts –reddened irregular elevated red patches and severe itching)

Investigations, management and ongoing assessment of anaphylaxis

ABCDE assessment

- Call for help – see Figure 4.3.
- Establish airway and commence CPR if necessary.
- Administer high flow 100% oxygen.
- Gain IV access and give fluids to maintain BP.
- Monitor (at a minimum):
  - pulse oximetry;
  - blood pressure;
  - 3-lead ECG.

- Position woman appropriately:
  - If she is conscious, sitting her up may improve her breathing.
  - If her blood pressure is low, lie her flat with tilt.
  - If she is unconscious but breathing, put her in the recovery position on the left side.

- Remove trigger:
  - Stop drugs, IVs (bloods, colloids, antibiotics);
  - Remove the stinger after a bee sting;
  - If food the suspected trigger, do not attempt to make the woman vomit.

Vital signs

Continued monitoring of respirations, oxygen saturations, pulse and blood pressure at a frequency determined by the woman's condition.

Fluid management

IV fluids will be maintained at a rate determined by the woman's condition, but care must be taken not to overload – strict records by the midwife are necessary.

Insertion of an indwelling urinary catheter will be undertaken as soon as possible to enable assessment of urinary output and accurate fluid balance records.

Drugs

Epinephrine (adrenaline) is the drug of choice in the management of anaphylaxis, and should be present on all emergency trolleys in a preloaded syringe. IM epinephrine (adrenaline) should be given immediately to all women with life-threatening symptoms.[21] Further drug therapy is an important part of treatment and may include IV epinephrine (this should be administered only by those trained to do so), antihistamines, corticosteroids and bronchodilators.

Investigations

Blood gases must be monitored and a full blood count, electrolyte assessment and clotting studies carried out.

Serial serum mast cell tryptase estimations are usually taken, as rise and fall will help with diagnosis.[27] The peak can occur between 30 minutes and 6 hours.

A 12-lead electrocardiograph (ECG) and X-ray may be required.

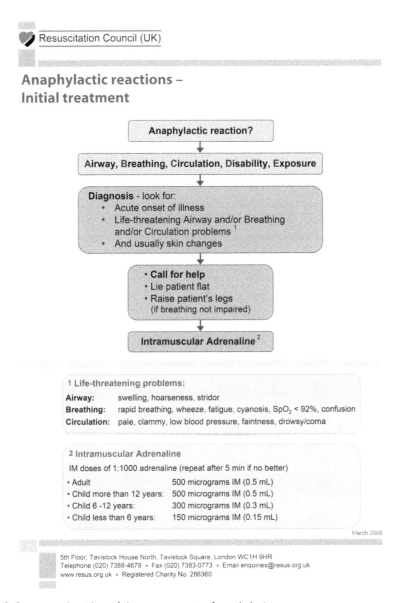

Resuscitation Council (UK)

**Anaphylactic reactions –
Initial treatment**

Anaphylactic reaction?

↓

Airway, Breathing, Circulation, Disability, Exposure

↓

Diagnosis - look for:
- Acute onset of illness
- Life-threatening Airway and/or Breathing and/or Circulation problems [1]
- And usually skin changes

↓

- **Call for help**
- Lie patient flat
- Raise patient's legs
  (if breathing not impaired)

↓

Intramuscular Adrenaline [2]

1 Life-threatening problems:

Airway: swelling, hoarseness, stridor
Breathing: rapid breathing, wheeze, fatigue, cyanosis, SpO_2 < 92%, confusion
Circulation: pale, clammy, low blood pressure, faintness, drowsy/coma

2 Intramuscular Adrenaline

IM doses of 1:1000 adrenaline (repeat after 5 min if no better)

- Adult   500 micrograms IM (0.5 mL)
- Child more than 12 years: 500 micrograms IM (0.5 mL)
- Child 6 -12 years: 300 micrograms IM (0.3 mL)
- Child less than 6 years: 150 micrograms IM (0.15 mL)

March 2008

5th Floor, Tavistock House North, Tavistock Square, London WC1H 9HR
Telephone (020) 7388-4678 • Fax (020) 7383-0773 • Email enquiries@resus.org.uk
www.resus.org.uk • Registered Charity No. 286360

Figure 4.3 Summary algorithm of the management of anaphylaxis

Source: Reproduced with the kind permission of the Resuscitation Council (UK)

Amniotic fluid embolism (anaphylactoid syndrome of pregnancy)

Amniotic fluid embolism (AFE) usually includes a sudden cardiovascular collapse, DIC (disseminated intravascular coagulation) and hypoxia, often manifesting as an altered mental state or respiratory arrest. In the UK and Ireland, at present AFE is the fifth most common cause of maternal mortality. Extensive recent research[28] covering 2005–14 has suggested a case fatality rate of 19% with significant long-term morbidity, including permanent neurological injury for many AFE survivors.

Out of the 23 women who died between 2005 and 2014,[28] the median time of death was 1 hour and 42 minutes after presentation of AFE. For all women with the diagnosis of AFE, 53% presented before or at the time of birth, the remainder presenting a median of 19 minutes after delivery. Most cases of AFE are associated with Caesarean section (71%) or an instrumental delivery (20%).[28,29] It is of course possible that these women had their deliveries expedited because of symptoms that were later diagnosed as AFE.

The pathophysiology of AFE is unclear. It seems that amniotic fluid may enter the maternal circulation without causing problems. However, in some women, an inflammatory response can develop, causing a rapid collapse similar to anaphylaxis or septic shock. Once amniotic fluid enters the maternal circulation there are thought to be a number of haemodynamic, humoral and coagulopathic changes that may occur and lead to the signs and symptoms of AFE. There is some evidence for the theory that an immunological mechanism is the major cause.[30] Despite the uncertainty of why the immune response occurs, it is clear that the effect on the woman can be devastating.

Clinical features

Signs and symptoms

The first symptoms seen may be shortness of breath and altered mental state, followed by cardiovascular collapse and DIC.[31] However, haemorrhage may be in the first symptom, or in some cases fetal bradycardia. Seizures are a less-common presenting symptom. Amniotic fluid embolism should always be suspected if a previously-asymptomatic healthy woman develops cardiac or respiratory failure during labour, Caesarean section or immediately after.

Analysis of the American Registry showed that the symptoms of women diagnosed with amniotic fluid embolism were as follows, given in the order in which they most commonly occurred:[32]

- Hypotension
- Fetal distress
- Pulmonary oedema
- Cardiopulmonary arrest
- Cyanosis
- Coagulopathy
- Respiratory distress

- Convulsions
- Uterine atony
- Bronchospasm.

In individual women, these symptoms can appear alone, in combination and of course in any order. Hypotension, hypoxia, DIC and/or altered mental state was present in 80–100% of affected women.[33] Diagnosis is made on clinical symptoms, after exclusion of other possible causes. UKOSS,[34] who have been monitoring AFE occurrences since 2005, define AFE clinically, using set criteria for diagnosis (see Box 4.9).

Box 4.9 UKOSS[34] case definition for AFE

Either: clinical diagnosis, such as maternal collapse with one or more of the following features: cardiac arrest, acute hypotension, acute hypoxia, cardiac arrhythmias, seizures, haemorrhage/coagulopathy, premonitory symptoms, sudden fetal compromise;

or: pathological diagnosis: the presence of fetal squames or hair in the lungs.
(In the absence of any other potential explanation for the signs and symptoms.)

Predisposing/risk factors

In the search to find some way to predict AFE, there have been many studies undertaken trying to identify predisposing and risk factors. However, the small number of women who suffer from AFE and the difficulty of diagnosis makes a definitive list challenging. See Box 4.10 for a list of possible risk factors.

Box 4.10 Possible risk factors for AFE[34,35,36,37]

- 'Tumultuous' contractions;*
- Age over 35 years (especially primiparous);
- Caesarean section;
- Assisted vaginal delivery;
- Induction of labour with prostaglandins or oxytocin;
- Augmentation with oxytocin;
- Artificial rupture of membranes;
- Woman has a medical history of allergy or atopy;[38]
- Multiple pregnancy/large fetus (uterine overdistension);
- Meconium;
- Long labour;
- Abruption/placenta praevia.

* It is possible that the reported tumultuous contractions are not the cause of the AFE, but a reaction to it.

Investigations, management and assessment of AFE

ABC assessment

Secure airway, assess respirations and administer oxygen or manually ventilate with an Ambu bag or intubation, depending on the site and availability of equipment or personnel. Pulse oximetry should be commenced to monitor respiratory function.

Cardiac massage is commenced if cardiac arrest has occurred. Two large-bore cannulae should be inserted as soon as possible, to support circulation and in anticipation of massive haemorrhage. An indwelling urinary catheter is inserted at the earliest opportunity. Fluids and/or blood products should be given according to the woman's needs. Note that because of the possibility of overloading the circulation, careful fluid balance is necessary.

Frequent monitoring of vital signs is necessary to assess the woman's condition. If still pregnant, peripartum Caesarean section may be necessary for successful resuscitation, and the midwife needs to anticipate this.

Assessment/prevention of coagulopathy

The uterine tone needs to be assessed almost constantly, as massive haemorrhage is so common, and the MOH protocol should be triggered if there is any indication of bleeding.[39]

Drugs such as oxytocin, ergometrine and prostaglandins will be used as necessary with surgical procedures (tamponade, brace suture) and bimanual compression is common. Hysterectomy has been reported in the literature to be necessary in about one quarter of women.[30]

Laboratory investigations

Clotting factors are assessed frequently, as well as FBC for levels of Hb and platelets. 'Bedside' tests may be used (see Chapter 5).

Electrolytes and ABG assessments are carried out to evaluate the renal and respiratory systems.

Chest X-rays, 12-lead ECGs, echocardiograms and lung V/Q scans may be carried out but no tests should delay basic, comprehensive and ongoing resuscitation. A previous Confidential Enquiries[40] noted sub-standard care in two cases when resuscitation was delayed as women were sent for unnecessary diagnostic scans.

Ongoing assessment

Most commonly, after an AFE the woman will initially be stabilised and then transferred to an intensive care facility for supportive care. Midwives will usually only care for this woman when she has been moved back to the maternity critical care unit, and it is likely her needs will mainly involve the same elements as women recovering from a massive haemorrhage (see Chapter 5).

Further reading

Resuscitation Council (UK). 2008. Emergency treatment of anaphylactic reactions: guidelines for healthcare providers. Available at www.resus.org.uk/anaphylaxis/emergency-treatment-of-anaphylactic-reactions/. Accessed 23 September 2017.

Rhodes, A, Evans, LE, Alhazzani, W, Levy, MM, Antonelli, M, Ferrer, R, Kumar, A . . . and Dellinger, RP. 2017. Surviving sepsis campaign: international guidelines for management of sepsis and septic shock: 2016. *Critical Care Medicine*, 45(3): 486–552.

Royal College of Obstetricians and Gynaecologists (RCOG). 2012a. Green-top guideline no. 64a: bacterial sepsis in pregnancy. London: RCOG. Available at www.rcog.org.uk/globalassets/documents/guidelines/gtg_64a.pdf. Accessed 20 March 2018.

Royal College of Obstetricians and Gynaecologists (RCOG). 2012b. Green-top guideline no. 64b: bacterial sepsis following pregnancy. London: RCOG. Available at www.rcog.org.uk/globalassets/documents/guidelines/gtg_64b.pdf. Accessed 20 March 2018.

Surviving sepsis campaign guidelines provide up-to-date guidance and educational resources for diagnosis, management and treatment of sepsis. Available at www.survivingsepsis.org/Guidelines/Pages/default.aspx.

References

1. Tait, D. 2012. The patient in shock. In: Tait, D, James, J, Williams, C and Barton, D (eds). *Acute and critical care in adult nursing*. London: Sage, pp. 122–46.

2. Paterson-Brown, S and Howell, C (eds). 2016. The MOET course manual: managing obstetric emergencies and trauma. Cambridge, UK: Cambridge University Press.

3. Vause, S, Clarke, B, Thomas, S, James, R, Lucas, S, Youd, E . . . and Knight, M on behalf of the MBRRACE-UK cardiovascular chapter writing group. 2016. Lessons on cardio-vascular disease. In: Knight, M, Nour, M, Tuffnell, D, Kenyon, S, Shakespeare, J, Brocklehurst, P and Kurinczuk, JJ (eds) on behalf of MBRRACE-UK. *Saving lives, improving mothers' care: surveillance of maternal deaths in the UK 2012–14 and lessons learned to inform maternity care from the UK and Ireland confidential enquiries into maternal deaths and morbidity 2009–14*. Oxford, UK: National Perinatal Epidemiology Unit, University of Oxford, pp. 33–68.

4. UK Sepsis Trust. 2016. Inpatient maternal sepsis tool kit. Available at https://sepsistrust.org/education/clinical-tools/. Accessed 16 September 2017.

5. National Institute for Health and Care Excellence. 2016. Sepsis: recognition, diagnosis and early management: NICE guideline [NG51]. Available at www.nice.org.uk/guidance/ng51. Accessed 16 September 2017.

6. Churchill, D, Rodger, A, Clift, J and Tuffnell, D on behalf of the MBRRACE-UK sepsis chapter writing group. 2014. Think sepsis. In: Knight, M, Kenyon, S, Brocklehurst, P, Neilson, J, Shakespeare, J and Kurinczuk, J (eds) on behalf of MBRRACE-UK. *Saving lives, improving mothers' care: lessons learned to inform future maternity care from the UK and Ireland confidential enquiries into maternal deaths and morbidity 2009–12*. Oxford, UK: National Perinatal Epidemiology Unit, University of Oxford, pp. 27–44.

7. Knight, M, Nour, M, Tuffnell, D, Kenyon, S, Shakespeare, J, Brocklehurst, P and Kurinczuk, JJ (eds) on behalf of MBRRACE-UK. 2016. *Saving lives, improving mothers' care: surveillance of maternal deaths in the UK 2012–14 and lessons learned to inform maternity care from the UK and Ireland confidential enquiries into maternal deaths and morbidity 2009–14*. Oxford, UK: National Perinatal Epidemiology Unit, University of Oxford.

8. Centre for Maternal and Child Enquiries (CMACE). 2011. Saving mothers' lives: reviewing maternal deaths to make motherhood safer: 2006–2008. The eighth report on confidential enquiries into maternal deaths in the United Kingdom. *British Journal of Obstetrics and Gynaecology*, *118*(1): s1–203.

9. Singer, M, Deutschman CS, Seymour CW, Shankar-Hari, M, Annane, D, Bauer, M . . . and Angus, DC. 2016. The third international consensus definitions for sepsis and septic shock (sepsis-3). *JAMA*, *315*(8): 801–10. doi: 10.1001/jama.2016.0287.

10. Bothamley, J. 2017. How to: recognise maternal sepsis. *Midwives*, 20(summer): 42–3.

11. Raynor, M. 2012. Sepsis. In: Raynor, M, Marshall, J and Jackson, K (eds). *Midwifery practice: critical illness, complications and emergencies case book*. Maidenhead, UK: McGraw Hill, pp. 175–92.

12. Bick, D, Beake, S and Pellowe, C. 2011. Vigilance must be a priority: maternal genital tract sepsis. *The Practising Midwife*, *14*(4): 16–18.

13. Bothamley, J and Boyle, M. 2015. *Infections affecting pregnancy and childbirth*. London: Radcliffe.

14. Lucas, DN, Robinson, PN and Nel, MR. 2012. Sepsis in obstetrics and the role of the anaesthetist. International Journal of Obstetric Anesthesia, 21(1): 56–67.

15. Acosta, C, Kurinczuk, J, Lucas, D, Tuffnell, D, Sellers, S and Knight, M. 2014. Severe sepsis in the UK, 2011–2012: a national case-control study. *PLoS Medicine*, *11*(7): e1001672. doi: 10.1371/journal.pmed.101672.

16. Acosta, CD and Knight, M. 2013. Sepsis and maternal mortality. *Current Opinion in Obstetrics and Gynecology*, *25*(2): 109–16.

17. Royal College of Obstetricians and Gynaecologists (RCOG). 2012a. Green-top guideline no. 64a: bacterial sepsis in pregnancy. London: RCOG. Available at www.rcog.org.uk/globalassets/documents/guidelines/gtg_64a.pdf.

18. Royal College of Obstetricians and Gynaecologists (RCOG). 2012b. Green-top guideline no. 64b: bacterial sepsis following pregnancy. London: RCOG. Available at www.rcog.org.uk/globalassets/documents/guidelines/gtg_64b.pdf.

19. Rhodes, A, Evans, LE, Alhazzani, W, Levy, MM, Antonelli, M, Ferrer, R, Kumar, A . . . and Dellinger, RP. 2017. Surviving sepsis campaign: international guidelines for management of sepsis and septic shock: 2016. *Critical Care Medicine*, *45*(3): 486–552.

20. UK Sepsis Trust. 2017. The sepsis six. Available at https://sepsistrust.org/education/. Accessed 16 September 2017.

21. Resuscitation Council (UK). 2008. Emergency treatment of anaphylactic reactions: guidelines for healthcare providers. Available at www.resus.org.uk/anaphylaxis/emergency-treatment-of-anaphylactic-reactions/. Accessed 23 September 2017.

22. Owen, JA, Punt, J and Stranford, SA. 2013. *Kuby immunology*. New York: WH Freeman and Company.

23. National Institute for Health and Care Excellence. 2011. Anaphylaxis: assessment and referral after emergency treatment: clinical guideline 134. Available at www.nice.org.uk/guidance/cg134/chapter/Introduction. Accessed 23 September 2017.

24. O'Connor, M, Smith, A, Nair, M, Fitzpatrick, K, Peiregalel, P, Kurinczuk, JJ and Knight, M. 2015. UKOSS annual report. Oxford, UK: National perinatal epidemiology unit.

25. Gibson, P and Powrie, R. 2011. Respiratory disease. In: James, D, Steer, P, Weiner, C, Gonik, B, Crowther, C and Robson, S (eds). *High risk pregnancy: management options*. St Louis, MO: Elsevier Saunders, pp. 657–82.

26. Camm, CF and Camm, AJ. 2016. *Clinical guide to cardiology*. Oxford, UK: Wiley-Blackwell.

27. Association of Anaesthetists of Great Britain and Ireland (AAGBI). 2009. Suspected anaphylactic reactions associated with anaesthesia. Available at www.aagbi.org/sites/default/files/anaphylaxis_2009.pdf. Accessed 23 September 2017.

28. Fitzpatrick, KE, Tuffnell, D, Kurinczuk, JJ and Knight, M. 2015. Incidence, risk factors, management and outcomes of amniotic-fluid embolism: a population-based cohort and nested case-control study. *British Journal of Obstetrics and Gynaecology*, *123*(1): 100–9. doi: 10.1111/1471–0528.13300.

29. Conde-Agudelo, A and Romero, R. 2009. Amniotic fluid embolism: an evidence-based review. *American Journal of Obstetrics and Gynecology*, *201*(5): 445.

30. Tuffnell, D and Slemeck, E. 2014. Amniotic fluid embolism. *Obstetrics, Gynaecology and Reproductive Medicine*, *24*(5): 148–52.

31. Stafford, I and Sheffield, J. 2007. Amniotic fluid embolism. *Obstetrics and Gynecology Clinics of North America*, *34*(3): 545–53.

32. Clark, S, Hankins, G, Dudley, DA, Dildy, GA and Porter, TF. 1995. Amniotic fluid embolism: analysis of the national registry. *American Journal of Obstetrics and Gynecology*, *172*(4, 1): 1158–69.

33. Rudra, A, Chatterjee, S, Sengupta, S, Nandi, B and Mitra, J. 2009. Amniotic fluid embolism. *Indian Journal of Critical Care Medicine*, *13*(3): 129–35.

34. Knight, M, McClymont, C, Fitzpatrick, K, Peirsegaele, P, Acosta, C, Spark, P and Kurinczuk, JJ on behalf of UKOSS. 2012. United Kingdom Obstetric Surveillance System (UKOSS) annual report 2012. Oxford, UK: National Perinatal Epidemiology Unit.

35. Abenhaim, H, Azoulay, L, Kramer, M and Leduc, L. 2008. Incidence and risk factors of amniotic fluid embolisms: a population-based study on 3 million births in the United States. *American Journal of Obstetrics and Gynecology*, *199*(1): 49.

36. Kramer, M, Rouleau, J, Baskett, T and Joseph, K on behalf of Maternal Health Study Group of the Canadian Perinatal Surveillance System. 2006. Amniotic-fluid embolism and medical induction of labour: a retrospective, population-based cohort study. *Lancet*, *368*(9545): 1444–8.

37. Kocarev, M and Lyons, G. 2007. Amniotic fluid embolism. In: Dob, D, Cooper, G and Holdcroft, A (eds). *Crises in childbirth: why mothers survive*. Oxford, UK: Radcliffe.

38. Hikiji, W, Tamura, N, Shigeta, A, Kanayama, N and Fukunaga, T. 2012. Fatal amniotic fluid embolism with typical pathohistological, histochemical and clinical features. *Forensic Science International*, *226*(1–3): e16–19.

39. Harper, A and Wilson, R on behalf of the MBRRACE-UK amniotic fluid embolism chapter writing group. 2014. Caring for women with amniotic fluid embolism. In: Knight, M, Kenyon, S, Brocklehurst, P, Neilson, J, Shakespeare, J and Kurinczuk, JJ (eds) on behalf of MBRRACE-UK. *Saving lives, improving mothers' care: lessons learned to inform future maternity care from the UK and Ireland confidential enquiries into maternal deaths and morbidity 2009–12*. Oxford, UK: National Perinatal Epidemiology Unit, University of Oxford, pp. 57–63.

40. Lewis, G, (ed.). 2007. The confidential enquiry into maternal and child health (CEMACH). Saving mothers' lives: reviewing maternal deaths to make motherhood safer 2003–2005. The seventh report on confidential enquiries into maternal deaths in the UK. London: CEMACH.

Haemorrhage

Introduction

Haemorrhage, both antenatal and postnatal, is probably one of the commonest causes for admission to a critical care unit. It remains a frequent cause of maternal mortality and, of course, long-term morbidity. Additionally, antepartum haemorrhage is responsible for the loss of many pregnancies, as well as for infant mortality/morbidity from premature delivery.

Physiology

Bleeding of any significant amount can result in hypovolaemic shock. In many ways, the woman's body is ready to deal with bleeding around childbirth; however, these compensatory mechanisms will begin to fail if bleeding is excessive or does not stop. The expansion of plasma volume in pregnancy and the efficiency of compensatory mechanisms mean that postnatal women may not show any signs of hypovolaemia, including a drop in BP, until they lose up to 1,500 ml of blood.[1] This means that, once signs and symptoms are obvious, the woman is already critically unwell.

When the woman starts to bleed, the circulating blood volume decreases and this causes the blood pressure to start to drop as the cardiac output falls. The fight or flight response of the sympathetic autonomic nervous system then immediately responds by producing adrenaline and noradrenaline, which increases the rate (tachycardia) and force of the heart's contraction and causes vasoconstriction (arterial and venous). Blood is diverted from non-vital areas such as the gastrointestinal (GI) tract and skin to maintain blood pressure to vital organs. The midwife may note that the woman looks pale and feels cold/clammy when her pulse is taken. The woman may say she feels nauseous. The liver and spleen add to the circulating volume by pushing stored red blood cells into the circulation and there is movement of interstitial fluid into the capillaries. The hypothalamus detects a loss of volume and this stimulates the release of anti-diuretic hormone (ADH) from the pituitary. In addition, the renin–angiotensin–aldosterone system causes reabsorption of sodium and water follows sodium. These mechanisms result in a decrease in the urine output as the body tries to conserve water and the woman may describe feeling thirsty. Hourly measurement of urine output is a helpful assessment in determining the extent of hypovolaemia and as an indication of recovery.

As hypovolaemia continues, the cells will switch to anaerobic metabolism, making adenosine triphosphate (ATP) (energy) without oxygen. This causes a build-up of lactic acid. The body responds by increasing the respiratory rate to try to blow off excess carbon dioxide.

An increase in heart rate is an early indication of compensation in hypovolaemic shock. Recognition of this will be particularly important in cases of concealed or persistent bleeding. Any amount of significant bleeding, or disruption of the clotting factors (as in the case of an intrauterine death) can lead to disseminated intravascular coagulation (DIC) (see Box 5.1).

However, although a maternal heart rate of over 100 warrants referral for close investigation, it is worth noting that bradycardia has been observed in cases of hypovolaemic shock. It is thought that parasympathetic nerve stimulation can be activated by the presence of blood clots in the cervix or from peritoneal irritation, creating an opposite of fight or flight response.[1]

Box 5.1 Disseminated intravascular coagulopathy (DIC)

DIC is secondary to other pathologies, causing uncontrolled systemic activation of coagulation alongside widespread clotting that leads to haemorrhage, hypotension, microvascular obstruction and necrosis, haemolysis and organ dysfunction.

Obstetric triggers include haemorrhage (particularly abruption), pre-eclampsia/eclampsia, HELLP syndrome, amniotic fluid embolism, massive infection and retention of a dead fetus.[2]

There is progression of the condition from early symptoms (mild hypoxia, dyspnoea, petechial bleeding, mucocutaneous bleeding, purpura, confusion, rashes and mottled cool skin)[3] to massive bleeding from multiple sites. It can be observed that blood seen does not clot.

Diagnosis is frequently done on clinical signs, but blood tests would include.

increased FDPs; increased soluble fibrin complexes; decreased fibrinogen; decreased platelets; prolonged clotting times.[2]

General predisposing/risk factors

It is acknowledged that many risk factors for both antepartum and postpartum haemorrhage exist, and serve as a trigger for midwives to ensure women give birth in appropriate environments, with skilled help and necessary equipment close at hand. However, it must always be remembered that, in many cases of both APH and PPH,[4] there are no identifiable risk factors.

Antepartum haemorrhage

Antepartum haemorrhage (APH) is defined by the RCOG as bleeding from or into the genital tract from 24 weeks of pregnancy and prior to the birth of the baby.[5] It is thought to complicate 3–5% of pregnancies.[5] The latest MBRRACE report[6] identified two women who died from abruption, and one from placenta praevia percreta.

Although it is known that the amount of blood visible is frequently not representative of the severity of the bleed, the RCOG[5] have divided APH into categories (see Box 5.2). However, it has often been noted that a small bleed precedes a large one, and for this reason women with even small amounts of bleeding are often admitted to antenatal wards (or critical care areas) for observation. Early delivery is frequently necessary to maintain the wellbeing of the mother, or for fetal compromise.

Box 5.2 Suggested classifications for APH[5]

- Spotting: staining, streaking or blood spotting noted on underwear or sanitary protection;
- Minor haemorrhage: blood loss less than 50 ml that has settled;
- Major haemorrhage: blood loss of 50–1,000 ml with no signs of clinical shock;
- Massive haemorrhage: blood loss greater than 1,000 ml and/or signs of clinical shock.

The types of APH are divided into:

- *Placental*: abruption (accidental haemorrhage) or placenta praevia (inevitable haemorrhage).
- *Antenatal bleeding of unknown origin* (ABUO).
- *Vasa praevia*: bleeding from the fetal umbilical vessel, which, as it is not maternal blood loss, will not impact on the woman's condition but may be fatal for the fetus, and is frequently hard to diagnose initially as it only presents as vaginal bleeding. Severe changes to the CTG pattern/FHR on auscultation, and a stable maternal condition, following rupture of membranes, should alert the midwife to the possibility of a vasa praevia.

APH clinical features

APH: predisposing/risk factors

Many predisposing/risk factors are similar for both placental abruption and placenta praevia, but some are specific for only one of these conditions.

- Advanced maternal age;
- Multiparity;
- Smoking;
- Cocaine and other drug abuse;

- Uterine abnormalities;
- Fibroids;
- Thrombophilia/taking therapeutic anticoagulants;
- Early pregnancy bleeding;
- Previous placenta praevia or abruption;
- Multiple pregnancy;
- Endometriosis;
- Chronic hypertension/pre-eclampsia (abruption);
- Pre-gestational diabetes (abruption);
- Uterine scarring, including previous CS (placenta praevia);
- Assisted conception (placenta praevia);
- Previous manual removal of the placenta (placenta praevia);
- Previous TOP (placenta praevia).

ACUTE FACTORS

- Sudden decompression: rupture of membranes in polyhydramnios or multiple pregnancy;
- Abdominal trauma;
- Inflammatory conditions: chorioamnionitis/premature rupture of membranes (PROM).

APH: signs and symptoms

The most obvious sign of haemorrhage is bleeding, and that will frequently be the reason the woman seeks professional care. However, as previously mentioned, the amount of blood seen may not be representative of the seriousness of the haemorrhage. As the BP will not react until a significant amount of blood is lost, the rises in pulse and respiration rate (and CTG observation) will be the main guides for the midwife, and these checks in particular need repeating as a trend will be valuable information. The woman may also appear shocked (cold, clammy extremities, pale), and the tone of the uterus is an important assessment (see below).

APH: investigations, management and ongoing assessment

ABC

- Airway: ensure a clear airway and position appropriately.
- Breathing: monitor respirations, attach pulse oximetry and give oxygen as indicated.
- Circulation: cannulate appropriately, commence fluids according to the woman's needs and monitor pulse and BP.

Observation of blood loss and assessment of pain

The amount of blood loss that can be seen is dependent on the cause of the APH. During a bleed from a placenta praevia, careful observation will probably result in a reasonably accurate estimation. However, during an abruption, some (or even all) bleeding can be retained behind the placenta (concealed), and therefore not be visible.[7]

During an APH it is advisable to record/save all soiled pads and linen, as well as trying to get an impression of the amount of blood loss before admission. Although the amount of estimated blood loss is probably not as important as clinical observation, routine 'pad checks' would be good practice.

If the bleeding is the result of an abruption, there is likely to be constant pain, sometimes very severe. There also may be intermittent contraction-like extremes in the pain. Alternatively, if the bleeding is from a placenta praevia, there is likely to be no pain.

Evaluation of the pregnancy

Assessment of the fetus, initially by listening to the fetal heart and then by continuous CTG recording, is important not only to establish the health of the fetus but also because a deterioration in the CTG is frequently an early finding when a woman's condition is worsening.

When assessed, the tone of the uterus may give some indication of the cause and/or severity of the APH. During an abruption, blood that is retained behind the uterus can be forced back into the myometrium, and in sufficient amounts will cause a 'couvelaire uterus' (feeling rigid/hard on abdominal palpation). Very often when a couvelaire uterus is identified, there has been sufficient blood loss to cause fetal distress, and urgent action is necessary.

If a placenta praevia is the cause of the bleeding, palpation of the fetus will demonstrate a high presenting part or perhaps an unstable lie. When an abruption is taking place, it may not be possible to feel the fetus due to a couvelaire uterus, or because it is too painful for the woman to tolerate a palpation.

Vital signs

- **Pulse and respiration rate:** increased due to blood loss but may be exacerbated by anxiety about her condition and fear for her baby.
- **Level of consciousness:** a change in behaviour is often a sign of hypoxia.
- **Blood pressure:** due to pregnancy compensation, the BP often remains within normal limits until the woman is significantly compromised.
- **Pulse oximetry:** usually a good indication of oxygenation, but accuracy may be compromised during a large blood loss (see Chapter 2).
- **Temperature:** infection can cause APH, so an important finding.
- **Capillary refill and skin assessment:** any compromise is a significant finding (see Chapter 2).

It is very important to undertake vital sign monitoring regularly and chart on MEOWS (or specialty critical care charts) to ensure subtle changes are identified early.

Blood tests

When a woman presents with bleeding, it is usual to undertake blood tests as part of the initial assessment. The range of blood tests will depend on the amount of blood loss, the condition of the woman (and fetus) and her history, but may include:

- FBC;
- clotting factors;
- group and save;
- U&Es
- renal and/or liver function tests;
- Kleihauer test if Rhesus negative.

Since a common outcome following a bleed in pregnancy is admission to an antenatal ward, the midwife needs to ensure blood tests are repeated as necessary – for example, a woman with placenta praevia may be an in-patient for many days, experiencing occasional small bleeds. It would be important to check her FBC and clotting factors regularly, especially as she could need an emergency Caesarean section at any time.

Ongoing assessment

Women who have suffered a severe APH will have delivery of their baby expedited, as the bleeding is unable to be controlled until the uterus is empty. Following delivery, it is usual to care for them in a critical care setting, and the ongoing monitoring of their condition by the midwife will include the same considerations described below for PPH.

Postpartum haemorrhage

Postpartum haemorrhage (PPH) is commonly defined as:

- *Primary*: > 500 ml or any amount which compromises the woman's condition, during the first 24 hours following childbirth, and
- *Secondary*: excessive bleeding after 24 hours until 12 weeks following childbirth, usually associated with retained products and/or infection.

The RCOG[8] divides PPH into minor (500–1,000 ml) or major (> 1,000 ml), and major can be subdivided into moderate (1,001–2,000 ml) or severe (> 2,000 ml). However, other classifications are frequently used in the literature. When a woman has a lower body mass (e.g., < 60 kg), it is likely that a lower level of blood loss may be clinically significant.[6]

Worldwide, PPH is the leading cause of maternal mortality,[9] and in UK is the third commonest cause of direct maternal deaths.[10]

The causes for PPH can be considered under the 'Four Ts':

- Tone: atonic uterus (the most common reason for PPH), frequently associated with prolonged first and second stage and/or an overstretched uterus;

- Tissue: retained placental tissue or clots, stopping the uterus from contracting;
- Trauma: cervical or vaginal lacerations (and haematoma formation), ruptured uterus;
- Thrombin: clotting anomalies.

In addition:

- The woman could display signs of haemorrhage with an internal bleed, such as subcapsular liver rupture seen in pre-eclampsia and HELLP syndrome,[11] or following an unknown accidental injury during an operative delivery.
- Any woman who has bled in excess of what is expected has the potential to have further blood loss due to a possible reduction in her clotting factors, so even a relatively minor PPH can become life-threatening unless careful observation for further bleeding and treatment is undertaken as necessary.

PPH clinical features

PPH: predisposing/risk factors

- Abnormalities of coagulation/taking therapeutic anticoagulants;
- APH;
- History of previous PPH;
- Pre-eclampsia;
- Intra-amniotic infection;
- Overdistension of uterus – for example, caused by polyhydramnios, multiple pregnancy or fetal macrosomia;
- Lack of progress in second-stage/prolonged labour;
- Episiotomy or lacerations of any tissue (e.g., cervix, vagina, perineum);
- General anaesthesia/uterine relaxants (e.g., magnesium sulphate and nifedipine);
- Functional/anatomic distortion of uterus;
- Bladder distension;
- Partial placenta accreta;
- Retained placenta, or retained products/blood clots;
- Uterine rupture;
- Uterine inversion;
- Intra-uterine death;
- Amniotic fluid embolism.

PPH: signs and symptoms

The most obvious sign of haemorrhage is bleeding, but this could be a sudden and sizable gush, or a more insidious trickle. As previously mentioned, the amount of blood seen may not be representative of the seriousness of the haemorrhage, as the woman may be retaining a significant amount within her uterus. Her pulse and respirations may rise, but the BP will not react in the early stages. The woman may also appear shocked (cold, clammy extremities, pale), and if this is out of proportion to the amount of blood seen, the possibility of internal bleeding should be considered.

PPH: investigations, management and ongoing assessment

A woman who is admitted to critical care following a major PPH needs careful observation, and may have received – or need – drug, mechanical and/or surgical interventions, the effects of which the midwife needs to evaluate.

Care during and following a haemorrhage will likely involve many of the actions described; however, it is noted that some elements (in particular drugs/dosages/administration) may vary slightly in some units. Midwives will be familiar with their local policies, especially since in most hospitals a yearly update on emergencies is required.

ABC

- Airway: ensure a clear airway and position appropriately.
- Breathing: monitor respirations, attach pulse oximetry and give oxygen as indicated.
- Circulation: cannulate appropriately, commence fluids according to the woman's needs and monitor pulse and BP.

Physical examination of uterus

Assessment of the uterus is a routine ongoing action by midwives caring for women during or after a PPH. The uterus will be assessed for position and tone during any routine check, and the initial action when observing an abnormal blood loss or tone would be uterine massage ('rub up a contraction'), which should not only improve the uterine tone, but also expel any clots that may be inhibiting a contracted uterus.

Bimanual compression may be necessary if haemorrhage is ongoing

Bimanual compression is achieved through one hand being inserted into the anterior fornix of the vagina and clenched, while the other hand externally gathers the fundus and pulls it forward, thereby pressing the walls of the uterus together (see Figure 5.1). Alternatively, bimanual compression can be done externally, by grasping the uterus with both hands and squashing it between them, but this is less likely to be effective.

Observation of blood loss

It is well known that visual estimation of peripartum blood loss is inaccurate,[8] although estimation can be improved by the use of blood collection drapes and/or weighing swabs, inco-pads, etc. However, it has been suggested that the exact volume of blood loss may not be as important as clinical signs and symptoms.[12]

In most cases of haemorrhage, although the loss may not be able to be accurately estimated, it is clear when the amount is a cause for concern. Nevertheless, concealed haemorrhage should not be forgotten, and the uterus can be a silent reservoir allowing blood to fill it without obvious external signs of excessive loss. There are also many causes of internal bleeding, including ruptured ectopic pregnancy, unidentified damage during a CS, splenic artery rupture, hepatic rupture, uterine rupture and significant

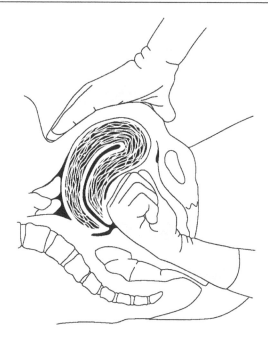

Figure 5.1 Bimanual compression
Source: Maureen Boyle. 2017. *Emergencies around childbirth*. Boca Raton, FL: CRC Press.

bleeding causing haematomas in the broad ligament or vagina. When vital signs (or complaints of pain) do not relate to the amount of blood seen, the midwife needs to be suspicious of concealed bleeding and be vigilant in abdominal palpation (establishing whether the uterus is high and/or rising) and whether abnormal pain during palpation is experienced. It may be necessary to add less-common observations (for example, regular girth measurements) to her assessments. A referral to obstetricians will usually result in evaluation by USS, but other tests or exploratory surgery may be necessary to establish a cause. However, the earlier the midwife can suspect a problem, and escalate her concerns, the better the outcome would be expected to be for the woman.

Maternal vital signs

The physiological increase in circulating blood volume during pregnancy means the signs of hypovolaemic shock become less sensitive in pregnancy.[8] It is thought that the pulse rate and particularly BP are usually maintained in the normal range until blood loss exceeds 1,000 ml, and only a slight recordable fall in systolic BP occurs with loss of 1,000–1,500 ml.[8]

- **Pulse and respiration rate:** increased due to blood loss but may be exacerbated by anxiety about her condition. Occasionally, despite blood loss, the pulse may remain within normal limits (see 'Physiology' section for an explanation).

- **Level of consciousness:** a change in behaviour is often a sign of hypoxia, but again may be influenced by her anxiety.
- **Blood pressure:** due to pregnancy compensation, the BP often remains within normal limits until the woman is very compromised. An arterial line may be used to give a continuous reading.
- **Pulse oximetry:** usually a good indication of oxygenation, but accuracy may be compromised during a large blood loss.[13]
- **Temperature:** infection can cause PPH, so an important finding.
- **Capillary refill and skin assessment:** any compromise is a significant finding.

CVP and arterial lines can provide important information and are commonly used following severe haemorrhage, but the threshold for their insertion is controversial. The responsibility lies with the senior anaesthetist, but ongoing monitoring will be undertaken by the midwife caring for the woman in critical care (see Chapter 2).

It is necessary to re-evaluate the woman's physiological condition frequently, even when bleeding appears to have stopped, to recognise if it continues or re-starts.[8] It is very important to undertake vital sign monitoring regularly and chart on MEOWS (or specialty critical care charts) to ensure subtle changes are identified early.

Blood tests

When a woman presents with bleeding, it is usual to undertake blood tests as part of the initial assessment. The range of blood tests will depend on the amount of blood loss, the condition of the woman and her history, but may include:

- FBC;
- clotting factors (PT, APTT, fibrinogen);
- group and save;
- cross match (usually 4 units minimum);
- U&Es;
- renal and/or liver function tests;
- lactate;
- ABGs.

As with many tests, these may be repeated and need to be carefully assessed, as the trends may be more valuable than a single measurement,[8] especially when the haemorrhage is not resolved, and, due to the time lapse, the findings available will only reflect the woman's condition when the blood was taken. The blood values aimed at during treatment are listed in Box 5.3.

Point-of-care testing has the advantage of immediate results, and includes the HemoCue system for haemoglobin estimation (< 1 minute) from a capillary sample, usually obtained from a fingertip skin puncture. However, some studies have shown poor agreement between laboratory and HemoCue results, particularly when using capillary blood and in the presence of oedema.[14] It might be expected that cold extremities may also have a compromising effect. Recommendations are that results should be viewed with caution and in relation to clinical observations.

Box 5.3 Main therapeutic aims post- (or during) haemorrhage[15]

- Hb > 80 g/l
- Platelet count > 50 × 10⁹/l
- PT (prothrombin time) < 1.5 times normal
- APTT (activated partial thromboplastin time) < 1.5 times normal
- Fibrinogen > 2 g/l

Measurements of serum lactate and base deficit (in conjunction with Hb/haematocrit) have been recommended by the European Society of Anaesthesiology[16] to assess oxygenation and tissue perfusion.

Thromboelastography (TEG^R) and rotational thromboelastometry (ROTEM^R)) are viscoelastic whole blood point-of-care testing devices that evaluate the haemostatic capacity of blood. Their use has been reported in the management of obstetric haemorrhage where, although they show the quality not quantity of platelets,[3] it could be valuable to identify those with low fibrinogen levels, and could help to individualise fibrinogen replacement.[16]

Although normal values in pregnancy and labour are only now being established, these devices may have a role in the management of blood product replacement in major obstetric haemorrhage. Laboratory findings have been found to correlate better with estimated blood loss, but TEG^R may be used as a conjunction to laboratory results, as it provides faster results.[17] At present, TEG^R and ROTEM^R are not recommended by NICE[18] for routine use.

Volume replacement

For all women who suffer a haemorrhage, fluid, especially blood and blood product replacements, will be routine management (see Chapter 3 for a discussion of these issues). MBRRACE-UK[6] have recently identified deaths where Hb measurements have falsely reassured staff, delaying transfusion, so it is important to treat with blood products according to clinical features, rather than necessarily wait for laboratory results.[8]

While fluid replacement is a vital part of the treatment of haemorrhage, and aggressive fluid resuscitation may be the initial response to hypotension, care must be taken not to dilute clotting factors further.[3] The midwife involved needs to ensure she is maintaining an accurate record of fluids infused, even in an emergency situation.

Current evidence suggests that crystalloids should only be used until the amount of blood loss becomes severe (approximately > 1,500 ml and/or symptoms of hypovolaemia).[19] Dilutional coagulopathy may occur when large volumes of crystalloid, colloid or RBC are used with insufficient transfusion of FFP and platelets: the recommendation is no more than 3.5 l of clear fluids, and early FFP should be considered for conditions with suspected coagulopathy, such as APH or AFE.[8]

See Chapter 3, section entitled 'Blood transfusion', for information on the various blood products, including FFP and cryoprecipitate, that will help correct coagulation disorders. Checking procedures to avoid transfusion errors and signs and symptoms of acute transfusion reactions are also discussed. Vital signs need to be recorded both before and within the first 15 minutes after transfusion begins.

Recommendations from the RCOG[8] as to fluid/blood transfusions are in Box 5.4.

Cell salvage (also known as autologous blood transfusion or intraoperative blood cell salvage) involves collection of the woman's own blood (via aspiration from the surgical field), then filtration, washing and reinfusion of red cells at the time a transfusion is needed.[1,20] The RCOG[8] suggest cell salvage should be considered for use when necessary for either Caesarean section or vaginal delivery. Initially, it was thought this procedure may lead to a risk of AFE, but this is no longer the case. However, fetal cells can enter the maternal circulation via this route, and therefore a Kleihauer test to check the size of fetal/maternal haemorrhage, and administration of an appropriate amount of anti-D, must be undertaken for Rh-negative women.

If a woman is bleeding from the genital tract, an indwelling urinary catheter will usually be inserted to ensure uterine contraction is not being compromised by a full bladder. In critical care environments, as well as during a major PPH, the catheter should have a urometer to enable monitoring of output.

Correction of electrolyte imbalance may be necessary, and this may include hyperkalaemia (secondary to high concentrations of potassium in transfused blood) and hypocalcaemia (chelated by the citrate found in transfused FFP).[21]

Recombinant factor VIIa (rFVIIa) may be used in cases of major haemorrhage. It achieves haemostasis by enhancing thrombin formation; however, it puts women at risk of thromboembolic events, so the presence of a senior haematologist is required. It only works if the woman has adequate platelets and fibrinogen, also necessary for clot generation.

Box 5.4 Fluid/blood product transfusion guidelines[8]

- Crystalloid: up to 2 l isotonic crystalloid.

- Colloid: up to 1.5 l colloid until blood arrives.

- Blood: if necessary, give group O, RhD-negative, K-negative red cell units (usually routinely kept on delivery suites for emergencies), and change to group-specific red cells as soon as available.

- FFP (fresh frozen plasma): given according to haemostatic testing (or 4 units FFP after 4 units of RBC) if haemorrhage is continuing.

- Platelet concentrations: 1 pool of platelets if platelet count $< 75 \times 10^9$/l and haemorrhage is continuing.

- Cryoprecipitate: 2 pools if fibrinogen < 2 g/l and haemorrhage is continuing.

Drugs

During a haemorrhage, pharmacological treatment is usually undertaken directly following or at the same time as uterine massage ('rubbing up a contraction'). Many of these drugs may also be used following a haemorrhage in critical care settings.

The RCOG[8] suggest:

- Oxytocin 5 iu slow IV (may repeat);
- Ergometrine 0.5 mg slow IV or IM (caution in women with hypertension);
- Oxytocin infusion 40 iu in 500 ml isotonic crystalloid at 125 ml/hour (if fluid restriction is necessary, a more concentrated solution can be made up with less fluid, and infused at a reduced rate);
- Carboprost (Hemabate) 0.25 mg IM, at intervals of > 15 minutes to a maximum of eight doses (caution in women with asthma);
- Misoprostol 800 micrograms SL (is frequently given PR).

In addition, tranexamic acid has been used extensively in medical conditions involving heavy blood loss, but its use in preventing PPH is relatively recent. Trials of its effectiveness and side-effects continue. It works by potentiating the blood clotting system as it is a fibrinolysis inhibitor.

Further midwifery considerations

THROMBOEMBOLIC

When recovering from a haemorrhage, women will have many risk factors for thromboembolic occurrence, and the midwife needs to ensure she encourages preventive measures,[22] especially since usual anticoagulant treatment may not be started immediately. Although early mobilisation would be ideal, it may not be possible, and therefore it is important to ensure:

- wearing of correctly-fitting anti-embolism stockings (AES);
- deep-breathing exercises to encourage venous return;
- effective post-partum pain relief to enable mobility;
- intermittent pneumatic compression devices used during operative procedures and while immobile;
- dehydration is identified (through the colour of the urine) and it is treated.

INFECTION

Infection rates are directly related to the length and the number of interventions during labour, and a woman who has haemorrhaged will have had many interventions. She is also likely to have some degree of anaemia, which is an important risk factor for infection. Besides making sure asepsis is followed wherever appropriate, the midwife could also ensure that the woman understands the importance of sleep and nutrition to efficient healing and building a healthy immune system.[23]

IMPORTANCE OF KEEPING WARM

It is important to avoid the vicious cycle of hypothermia, acidosis and coagulopathy in the woman who has suffered a massive haemorrhage. Warmed fluids must be given, and care directed to achieving normothermia by the use of devices such as forced air warmers.[21]

PSYCHOLOGICAL AND SOCIAL

If a woman has suffered a haemorrhage, it is likely to have been a frightening and possibly traumatic event. If the health of the baby was compromised this would have added to the psychological impact. Besides being a source of information and empathetic care, the midwife needs to ensure this woman knows how to access help if she feels the need after she returns home.

Additional interventions for postpartum haemorrhage

The recent fall in the rate of hysterectomy[24] as a treatment for PPH demonstrates that several advanced procedures have been introduced that have successfully managed the PPH while potentially conserving fertility. These will all involve medical specialists in the actual procedure, but it is likely that the midwife will be caring for the woman directly post-procedure and therefore needs an understanding of what was done, plus possible complications and monitoring required. It is also relevant to note that, while stopping the haemorrhage will obviously have been the priority, the bleeding may not have initially been caused by common obstetric reasons. In one analysis of outcomes of pelvic arterial embolisation, it was noted that, following successful treatment of the haemorrhage, some women progressed to hepatic failure or cardiomyopathy,[25] which suggests that these were probably the initial causes of the haemorrhage. Therefore, all midwifery assessments for women following haemorrhage treatment need to be underpinned by the suspicion that there may also be other pathologies present.

Pelvic artery embolisation

Selective uterine artery embolisation has proven to be a viable treatment for PPH, with studies showing a > 80% success rate.[25] The femoral artery is catheterised, and an initial aortogram identifies the relevant bleeding vessel by the use of a contrast medium. Occlusion of the vessel can be with absorbable or non-absorbable material, and a repeat angiogram is then done to confirm the success of the procedure.

However, the disadvantage to this treatment is that there needs to be accessible equipment and an available interventional radiologist to undertake the procedure.

When caring for a woman following pelvic arterial embolisation, it is usual to ensure she lies flat for several hours afterwards. She may also need pain medication, as uterine pain is frequently reported, and nausea, vomiting and/or a low-grade pyrexia should be treated. Ongoing assessment is necessary to ensure these symptoms and any others are monitored, and escalated if there is any cause for concern. Routine vital signs and blood loss must of course be frequently assessed.

Balloon tamponade

Balloon tamponade is considered by the RCOG[8] as an appropriate first-line 'surgical' intervention to treat uterine atony. Various types of hydrostatic balloon catheters are available. Rusch balloons may be most commonly-used, as they have a larger capacity, are easy to use and low-cost.[8]

With the woman usually in lithotomy position in theatre, and following appropriate anaesthesia, the balloon catheter is inserted under direct vision, with the aid of sponge-holding forceps.[26] An appropriate amount of warmed saline solution (depending on the type of balloon – usually 300–1,000 ml) is used to fill the balloon until resistance is felt. The vagina is then usually packed to ensure the balloon does not fall through the cervix. An indwelling urinary catheter is necessary, although it is likely that one is already in place following the haemorrhage.

When caring for a woman, the midwife needs to make sure she is aware of any internal packs/swabs and communicates this to other staff as appropriate. It would be good practice to routinely identify any woman with an internal pack in place – some units will do this by way of a distinctly coloured wristband which will be left on the woman until the pack is removed.

The balloon is left in for 12–48 hours – the timing will depend on individual circumstances. During this time, the midwife will monitor vital signs and observe frequently for bleeding. It is usual to maintain an IV syntocinon infusion, although this may be at a reduced concentration and/or rate. IV antibiotics will be prescribed.

Removal of the balloon should only take place when there are appropriate personnel available (and the woman is fasting) in case of resumed bleeding,[27] which may necessitate a return to theatre. Fluid is drained from the balloon gradually, usually at a rate of 100 ml every 15 minutes.[27] Continued observation for bleeding and of vital signs are maintained as long as appropriate.

Haemostatic compression (brace) suture

The use of a compression suture necessitates the uterus to be exposed, either through Caesarean section incision or laparotomy, and will be done in theatre, usually under a general anaesthetic. The aim is to exert a mechanical compression of the uterine vascular sinuses.[28] The methods vary, and can involve hysterotomy (B-Lynch) or remain external to the uterine cavity (modified compression suture).

Following the procedure, the midwife may care for the woman recovering from a GA, with the potential complications that may entail, and must continue to monitor for blood loss continuing or re-starting, by vital signs and observation. IV antibiotics will be prescribed.

Arterial balloon occlusion of the internal iliac arteries

Balloon catheters can be placed in the internal iliac arteries via the common femoral artery as an emergency measure to stop a massive PPH.[29] They can also be sited (with the balloons left uninflated) during preparation for a Caesarean section with a high risk of massive PPH, for example in the presence of placenta percreta. The balloons are usually deflated after 24 hours and removed after 48 hours.[29] Antibiotic prophylaxis is usual.

Surgical tying-off of arteries

Uterine artery ligation, utero-ovarian artery anastomosis or internal iliac artery ligation can be carried out. Following the surgery, the midwife will undertake the usual monitoring. There is a risk of internal bleeding with no visible blood loss evident, and therefore observations, documented on a MEOWS chart, are essential to identify compensatory signs of blood loss.

Hysterectomy

Despite recommendations that hysterectomy should be considered early in a severe PPH, particularly if associated with placenta accreta or uterine rupture,[8] hysterectomy is often the 'last resort' treatment. Therefore, when this woman is transferred to critical care, the midwife must be aware that she may have been severely compromised, perhaps for some time, and ensure she remains under very close observation for probably a considerable time.

Following the surgery, which is usually performed under general anaesthetic, the midwife may need to undertake appropriate observations while the woman is recovering from surgery, and maintain frequent comprehensive vital sign monitoring as well as observing for any blood loss.

Further reading

Mavrides, E, Allard, S, Chandraharan, E, Collins, P, Green, L, Hunt, BJ, . . . and Thomson, AJ on behalf of the Royal College of Obstetricians and Gynaecologists (RCOG). 2016. Green-top guideline no. 52 for PPH: prevention and management of postpartum haemorrhage. *British Journal of Obstetrics and Gynaecology, 124*(5): 106–49.

Royal College of Obstetricians and Gynaecologists (RCOG). 2011. Green-top guideline no. 63: antepartum haemorrhage. London: RCOG.

Royal College of Obstetricians and Gynaecologists (RCOG). 2011. Green-top guideline no. 56: maternal collapse in pregnancy and the puerperium. London, RCOG.

Royal College of Obstetricians and Gynaecologists (RCOG). 2011. Green-top guideline no. 27: placenta praevia, placenta praevia accreta and vasa praevia: diagnosis and management. London: RCOG.

References

1. Paterson-Brown, S and Howell, C. 2014. *Managing obstetric emergencies and trauma: the MOET course manual.* Cambridge, UK: Cambridge University Press.
2. Nelson-Piercy, C. 2015. *Handbook of obstetric medicine.* Boca Raton, FL: CRC Press.
3. Woodrow, P. 2012. *Intensive care nursing.* London: Routledge.
4. World Health Organisation (WHO). 2012. *WHO recommendations for the prevention and treatment of postpartum haemorrhage.* Geneva: WHO.
5. Royal College of Obstetricians and Gynaecologists (RCOG). 2011. Green-top guideline no. 63: antepartum haemorrhage. London: RCOG.

6. Paterson-Brown, S and Bamber, J on behalf of the MBRRACE-UK haemorrhage chapter writing group. 2014. Prevention and treatment of haemorrhage. In: Knight, M, Kenyon, S, Brocklehurst, P, Neilson, J, Shakespeare, J and Kurinczuk, JJ (eds) on behalf of MBRRACE-UK. *Saving lives, improving mothers' care: surveillance of maternal deaths in the UK 2012–14 and lessons learned to inform maternity care from the UK and Ireland confidential enquiries into maternal deaths and morbidity 2009–14.* Oxford, UK: National Perinatal Epidemiology Unit, University of Oxford, pp. 45–55.

7. Acosta, L. 2017. Antepartum haemorrhage. In: Boyle, M (ed.). *Emergencies around childbirth: a handbook for midwives.* Boca Raton, FL: CRC Press

8. Mavrides, E, Allard, S, Chandraharan, E, Collins, P, Green, L, Hunt, BJ, . . . and Thomson, AJ on behalf of the Royal College of Obstetricians and Gynaecologists (RCOG). 2016. Green-top guideline no. 52 for PPH: prevention and management of postpartum haemorrhage. *British Journal of Obstetrics and Gynaecology, 124*(5): 106–49.

9. Say, L, Chou, D, Gemmill, A, Tunçalp, O, Moller, A-B, Daniels, J . . . and Alkema, A. 2014. Global causes of maternal death: a WHO systematic analysis. *Lancet Global Health, 2*(6): 323–33.

10. Knight, M, Kenyon, S, Brocklehurst, P, Neilson, J, Shakespeare, J and Kurinczuk, JJ (eds) on behalf of MBRRACE-UK. Saving lives, improving mothers' care: surveillance of maternal deaths in the UK 2012–14 and lessons learned to inform maternity care from the UK and Ireland confidential enquiries into maternal deaths and morbidity 2009–14. Oxford, UK: National Perinatal Epidemiology Unit, University of Oxford.

11. Williamson, C and Girling, J. 2011. Hepatic and gastrointestinal disease. In: James, D, Steer, PJ and Weiner, CP (eds). *High risk pregnancy management options.* St Louis, MO: Elsevier Saunders, pp. 839–60.

12. Weeks, A and Mallaiah, S. 2016. Beyond MBRRACE: new developments to stem the tide of postpartum haemorrhage. *European Journal of Obstetrics and Gynecology and Reproductive Biology, 199*(April): 66–8.

13. Casey, G. 2001. Oxygen transport and the use of pulse oximetry. Nursing Standard, 15(47): 46–53.

14. Seguin, P, Kleiber, M, Chanavaz, C, Morcet, J and Mallédant, Y. 2011. Determination of capillary hemoglobin levels using the HemoCue system in intensive care patients. *Journal of Critical Care, 26*(4): 423–7.

15. Hunt, B, Allard, S, Keeling, D, Norfolk, D, Stanworth, SJ and Pendry, K on behalf of the British Committee for Standards in Haematology. 2015. A practical guideline for the haematological management of major haemorrhage. *British Journal of Haematology, 170*(6): 788–803.

16. Kozek-Langenecker, S, Afshari, A, Albaladejo, P, Aldecoa, C, Barauskas, G, De Robertis, E . . . and Zacharowski, K. 2013. Management of severe perioperative bleeding: guidelines from the European Society of Anaesthesiology. *European Journal of Anaesthesiology, 30*(6): 270–382.

17. Karlsson, O, Jeppsson, A and Hellgren, M. 2014. Major obstetric haemorrhage: monitoring with thromboelastography, laboratory analyses or both? *International Journal of Obstetric Anesthesia, 23*(1): 10–17.

18. National Institute for Health and Care Excellence (NICE). 2014. Detecting, managing and monitoring haemostasis: viscoelastometric point-of-care testing (ROTEM, TEG and Sonoclot systems). *NICE diagnostics guidance, 13.* Available at www.nice.org.uk/guidance/dg13.

19. Schorn, M and Phillippi, J. 2014. Volume replacement following severe postpartum hemorrhage. *Journal of Midwifery and Women's Health, 59*(3): 336–43.

20. Goucher, H, Wong, C, Patel, S and Toledo, P. 2015. Cell salvage in obstetrics. *Anesthesia and Analgesia, 121*(2): 465–8.

21. Jennings, A, Brunning, J and Brennan, C. 2012. Management of obstetric haemorrhage. *Anaesthesia tutorial of the week 257*. Available at www.frca.co.uk/Documents/257%20 Management%20of%20Obstetric%20Haemorrhage.pdf.
22. Bothamley, J. 2017. Thromboembolism in pregnancy. In: Boyle, M (ed.). *Emergencies around childbirth*. Boca Raton, FL: CRC Press, pp. 55–76.
23. Bothamley, J and Boyle, M. 2015. *Infections affecting pregnancy and childbirth*. London: Radcliffe.
24. Lennox, C and Marr, L on behalf of Reproductive Health Programme, Healthcare Improvement Scotland. 2014. Scottish confidential audit of severe maternal morbidity: reducing avoidable harm. 10th annual report. Edinburgh, UK: Healthcare Improvement Scotland.
25. Cheong, JY, Kong, TW, Son JH, Won, JH, Yang, JI and Kim, HS. 2014. Outcome of pelvic arterial embolization for postpartum hemorrhage: a retrospective review of 117 cases. *Obstetrics and Gynecology Science*, 57(1): 17–27.
26. Majumdar, A, Saleh, S, Davis, M, Hassan, I and Thompson, AJ. 2010. Use of balloon catheter tamponade for massive postpartum haemorrhage. *Journal of Obstetrics and Gynaecology*, 30(6): 586–93.
27. Keriakos, R, and Mukhopadhyay, A. 2006. The use of the Rusch balloon for management of severe postpartum haemorrhage. *Journal of Obstetrics and Gynaecology*, 26(4): 335–8.
28. Fotopoulou, C and Dudenhausen, J. 2010. Uterine compression sutures for preserving fertility in severe postpartum haemorrhage: an overview 13 years after the first description. *Journal of Obstetrics and Gynaecology*, 30(4): 339–49.
29. Penninx, J, Pasmans, H and Oei, S. 2010. Arterial balloon occlusion of the internal iliac arteries for treatment of life-threatening massive postpartum haemorrhage: a series of 15 consecutive cases. *European Journal of Obstetrics and Gynecology and Reproductive Biology*, 148(2): 131–4

Chapter 6

Pre-eclampsia (PET)

Introduction

Along with haemorrhage, pre-eclampsia and associated conditions (eclampsia, HELLP and AFLP) are likely to be the conditions midwives will most commonly care for in a critical care situation. These conditions present challenges for midwifery assessment due to the difficulties in identifying those at risk, a variety of presenting signs and symptoms, the unpredictable speed of the progression of disease and variations in response to treatment.

The basic definition for pre-eclampsia has traditionally been: new hypertension presenting after 20 weeks with significant proteinuria. However, in recognition of the multisystem effect PET has, the International Society for the Study of Hypertension in Pregnancy (ISSHP)[1] agreed a revised definition of pre-eclampsia in 2014. They defined pre-eclampsia as hypertension developing after 20 weeks gestation and the co-existence of one or more of the following new onset conditions: proteinuria, other maternal organ dysfunction (renal, liver, neurological, haematological complications) or utero-placental dysfunction (fetal growth restriction).

This revised international definition acknowledges PET as a multisystem disorder. The midwife therefore needs to be familiar with all possible symptoms of PET and recognise these in women with or without high BP or proteinuria. Follow-up examinations and blood and urine tests will aim to determine the presence of any of the signs of PET. Box 6.1 lists signs and symptoms associated with PET.

The most recent MBRRACE-UK[2] report has identified that deaths from hypertensive disorders are at the lowest ever rate, and consider that research, audit and evidence-based guidelines have led to this improvement. In the MBRRACE-UK[3] analysis of hypertensive disease, intracranial haemorrhage resulting from PET continued to be

---

Box 6.1 Signs and symptoms of pre-eclampsia

- Rise in BP (see Box 6.2 for NICE classification of BP);
- Proteinuria/oliguria;
- Development of epigastric or right upper quadrant pain/pain below the ribs/liver tenderness;
- Nausea and vomiting;
- Cerebral disturbances (headache, altered consciousness);
- Visual field disturbances (including blurred vision, flashing lights);
- Progressive oedema (frequently can be easily observed on the woman's face/hands);
- Abnormal renal function tests;
- Abnormal liver enzymes;
- Bleeding tendency: platelet count decreasing and/or clotting factors abnormality;
- Abnormalities in fetal assessment, including IUGR, reduced liquor volume and/or CTG recording (in some cases restriction of growth can precede the woman's symptoms).

Box 6.2 NICE[4] categories of hypertension

- Mild: diastolic 90–99 mmHg, systolic 140–149 mmHg;
- Moderate: diastolic 100–109 mmHg, systolic 150–159 mmHg;
- Severe: diastolic > 110, systolic > 160.

---

the most common cause of death, followed by hepatic complications. However, no women died in relation to inappropriate fluid management (pulmonary oedema and renal failure),[3] confirming that strict fluid restriction policies appear to be effective.

Nevertheless, there is no room for complacency when dealing with PET and associated conditions, as analysis of individual cases[3] has identified many areas where improvement to care may have made a difference to the outcome.

Physiology

The aetiology of pre-eclampsia remains unknown, but understanding has been advanced in recent years by scientists, and evidence is becoming increasingly available that the various theories presented have some common features. In a healthy pregnancy uncomplicated by pre-eclampsia, trophoblastic cells invade the maternal uterine arteries at both the decidual and myometrial level, resulting in erosion of the muscle layer and enlargement of the lumen. Additionally, there is increased synthesis of prostacyclin, nitric oxide and thromboxane A2, which create a change in homeostatic balance, with a tendency to vasodilatation of the uterine arteries. This results in lowered resistance in the arteries, absence of maternal vasomotor control and a substantial increase in blood supply to the placenta to meet the demands of the developing fetus. The associated changes account for the transient lowering of maternal blood pressure seen in early pregnancy, which is then compensated for by the physiologic increase in circulating blood volume.

The changes seen in pre-eclampsia appear to be caused by a complex interplay of abnormal genetic, immunological and placental factors.[5] The early changes in the way the placenta embeds in the uterus is considered to be significant, in that trophoblastic invasion of the placental bed spiral arteries is confined to the decidual level. As a consequence of this arrested trophoblastic invasion, adrenergic nerve supplies to the uterine spiral arteries are not disrupted, systemic vascular resistance remains high and placental perfusion is poor. The resultant effect is tissue hypoxia, which is believed to cause liberation of substances that are toxic to endothelial cells.[6,7] It has been suggested that this involves an inflammatory response,[6] and this damage to endothelial cells underlies the varied multi-organ dysfunction seen in PET.

The total peripheral vascular resistance increases in pre-eclampsia (as contrasted with the reduction expected in a normal pregnancy), and this is one of the causes of raised blood pressure. In addition, enhanced contraction of damaged blood vessels facilitates aggregation of platelets at the site of injury and may predispose to problems with coagulation.

In the kidneys, glomerular capillary endothelial swelling occurs accompanied by deposits of fibrinogen within and under the endothelial cells. This results in the general renal function being impaired, causing rising serum creatinine, uric acid and urea levels. In addition, increased glomerular permeability allows protein to escape into the urine.

The hypoalbuminemia of pre-eclampsia causes a lower colloid osmotic pressure, affecting fluid transport across the capillaries and resulting in too much fluid in the interstitial spaces (oedema) and too little in the vascular compartment (hypovolaemia). In addition to the cardiovascular and renal affects described above, reduced organ perfusion in the liver, pulmonary system and brain can contribute to the serious and potentially fatal outcomes seen in pre-eclampsia.

Clinical features

Predisposing/risk factors

Although it is acknowledged that pre-eclampsia is a very unpredictable disease and may occur in those with no predisposing factors, it can be useful to identify those at increased risk of developing this condition (see Box 6.3).

Many suggestions have been made regarding methods to specifically identify women who are at high risk of pre-eclampsia and would benefit from increased monitoring.[8] These include early blood tests, Doppler assessment of uterine blood flow and other procedures. However, although many assessments look promising, at present NICE have not recommended any of these tests for routine use.

Other conditions apart from those identified by NICE[4] (Box 6.3) have also been mentioned in the literature. Involvement of the father, such as second or subsequent pregnancy with a new partner[9] and women with partners who previously fathered a

---

Box 6.3 Women at risk of developing pre-eclampsia[4]

High risk:

- hypertensive disease during a previous pregnancy;
- chronic kidney disease;
- autoimmune disease, such as systemic lupus erythematosus or antiphospholipid syndrome;
- Type 1 or Type 2 diabetes;
- chronic hypertension.

Moderate risk:

- first pregnancy;
- age 40 years or older;
- pregnancy interval of more than 10 years;
- BMI of 35 kg/m^2 or more at first visit;
- family history of pre-eclampsia;
- multiple pregnancy.

---

baby resulting from a pregnancy with pre-eclampsia,[10,11] as well as a pregnancy involving donor material,[9] have been cited. The presence of abnormal placental material such as hydatidiform mole, or other anomalies such as hydrops fetalis or polyhydramnios, are also considered risk factors for pre-eclampsia.[12] Multiple pregnancy has long been accepted as a risk factor for pre-eclampsia, but recent research has suggested that DC (dichorionic) twin pregnancies are at even more risk than MC (monochorionic) twin pregnancies.[13]

A study comparing risk factors for early onset (< 34 weeks) pre-eclampsia with those for late onset (≥ 34 weeks) pre-eclampsia, found younger maternal age, nulliparity and diabetes mellitus were more strongly associated with late onset pre-eclampsia.[14]

Investigations, management and ongoing assessment of PET

Pre-eclampsia is an unpredictable disease and changes associated with a worsening condition do not necessarily follow a logical, sequential or linear progression. Some women may have a very severe presentation of pre-eclampsia where it could be anticipated eclampsia may be imminent, but eclampsia does not happen. Alternatively, some women first diagnosed with mild or moderate signs and symptoms can become severely ill in a very short period of time. Therefore, midwives must be alert for subtle changes, such as symptoms and trends in blood values/vital signs, to identify early a woman whose condition is deteriorating. A gradual deterioration in any of the signs and symptoms listed in Box 6.1 would indicate fulminating or worsening pre-eclampsia.

The main aims are to:

- control blood pressure to prevent strokes;
- restrict fluids to prevent pulmonary oedema;
- consider anticonvulsant therapy with magnesium sulphate to prevent eclampsia;
- identify any fetal compromise;
- plan delivery for the optimum time.

Therefore, awareness of these aims determines the testing and observations necessary for early detection of deterioration (impending seizure, organ failure, and/or pulmonary oedema). Continued assessment of vital signs, analysis of symptoms, physical examination and bloods will be maintained at intervals according to the woman's condition.

ABC

- Airway: ensure a clear airway and position appropriately.
- Breathing: monitor respirations, attach pulse oximetry and give oxygen as indicated.
- Circulation: cannulate appropriately, and monitor pulse and BP.

Vital signs

Blood pressure

Underpinning monitoring and treatment of pre-eclampsia are regular and frequent blood pressure measurements. These may range from as often as every 5 minutes, for a period of time when concern is high, to less frequently. However, the 'routine' regular measurements will only be a minimum – the midwife will undertake a blood pressure measurement whenever it is felt necessary, for instance if the woman reports new symptoms or the CTG interpretation changes. Blood pressure readings will underpin management of medication, so a recording before and at a suitable interval (depending on the drug) following anti-hypertensive administration will provide valuable information to ensure the correct drug, dose and timing are being offered.

Blood pressure can be taken with an automated machine, and in fact the lack of observer error and the assured regularity of the test will give an automated machine the advantage in producing an accurate trend during frequent measurement. However, there have been reported issues with automated machines, in particular under-reading, and most units will have a protocol for undertaking manual blood pressure recording: for instance, once a shift, or every 4 hours.

An arterial line (see Chapter 2) may be inserted to enable continuous monitoring of blood pressure, which will be displayed on a monitor. The arterial line will also allow easy access for arterial blood gas sampling.

Other vital signs

The midwife should note all vital signs (at a frequency determined by individual condition), with particular attention being paid not only to blood pressure but also to respirations, oxygen saturation readings, pulse and level of consciousness. Continuous oxygen saturation monitoring (see Chapter 2) may give an early warning of the onset of pulmonary oedema.

Recording blood pressure readings, together with other vital signs and assessments, on a MEOWS chart may allow trends to be identified as early as possible and enable interventions that may limit the occurrence of complications. However, MEOWS charts may not clearly identify subtle changes (especially when the BP is being successfully controlled with anti-hypertensives), and also rarely address some of the important signs and symptoms of PET, so the midwife must be alert to note these and appreciate their potential importance.

Blood tests

Blood for PET screening (see Box 6.4) will be done regularly, depending on the woman's condition, and recorded carefully in order to see the trend and hence assess the progress of the disease. Walker[15] suggests that a falling platelet count could be used as a guide to the timing of delivery, as it is associated with a worsening of the maternal and fetal condition. Adhesion of platelets to damaged endothelial blood vessel walls narrows the lumen, reduces end organ perfusion, exacerbates tissue damage through anoxia and predisposes the woman to development of eclampsia, placental abruption and possible fetal demise.

Box 6.4 PET screening blood

While many tests may be undertaken, of particular importance are:

- Full blood count
- Renal function tests
- Liver function tests.

Clotting studies may also be carried out. Blood may also be sent for 'group and save', as the likelihood of an imminent Caesarean section is high.

Fluid balance

Fluid management is vital to the successful management of pre-eclampsia. The importance of meticulous recording and evaluation of input and output cannot be over-emphasised. There have been no reported deaths from pulmonary causes in women with pre-eclampsia since the early 2000s, and this has been attributed to successful fluid restriction policies.[16]

All maternity unit policies for pre-eclampsia care will contain a section regarding fluid restriction, and midwives will need to remember that IV infusions, bolus drug infusions and oral intake should be included in the 'allowed' (usually about 80 ml/hour) amount of fluid.[4]

Although proteinuria is often caused by a urinary tract infection (and a MSU for MC&S should always be sent), it is also possible that it may be the first sign of pre-eclampsia in a woman with normal blood pressure. The reagent strips ('dipsticks') commonly used in clinical practice should be considered a guide only to the presence of protein in the urine and not be accepted as an accurate quantification of protein excretion. When evaluating proteinuria, a urine specimen for urinary spot protein: creatinine ratio (PCR) is commonly used. Dependent on local policy, action may be taken on the PCR result, or a 24-hour urinary collection may be necessary.[17] Results of more than 30 mg/mmol for the PCR and more than 300 mg in a 24-hour collection are considered significant and therefore abnormal.[4]

It should be remembered that the quantity of protein present in urine samples may not be indicative of renal damage, but instead may be a reflection of capillary leakage and more accurately a projection of the development of generalised oedema. Where protein loss is significant, the possibility of pulmonary and/or cerebral oedema as complications of pre-eclampsia is considerable.

In most women hospitalised with moderate to severe pre-eclampsia, an indwelling urinary catheter will be used and the urine measured hourly (output should be 0.5 ml/kg/hr and should not fall below 30 ml/hr or 100 ml/4 hourly). It may be tested for the quantity of protein. If the woman has given birth and had a PPH (not an uncommon scenario), fluid management is a particular challenge. As a very fine balance between intake and output is required, this may be best achieved by monitoring via a central venous pressure (CVP) line (see Chapter 2), to underpin fluid management. Careful records must be kept of fluid balance. See Chapter 3 for further discussion of this important subject.

Drugs

The aim of anti-hypertensive treatment is usually to keep the systolic blood pressure below 150 mmHg and the diastolic blood pressure between 80 and 100 mmHg,[4,18] which is thought to be a safe compromise as further reductions may well impair placental perfusion and affect fetal wellbeing.

Ongoing evaluation is necessary to identify signs and symptoms (see Box 6.5) that may lead to eclampsia or organ failure. Magnesium sulphate (see 'Eclampsia' section in this chapter) is usually prescribed to prevent eclampsia if a woman has severe hypertension and proteinuria or mild-to-moderate hypertension and proteinuria, with one or more of the related signs and symptoms.[4]

Fetal assessment

Careful fetal assessment is undertaken, as any deterioration may indicate a change in the woman's condition, as well as a compromised fetus. This may include bio-physical assessment by ultrasound to establish growth, determine the degree of hypoxaemia and fetal reserve (via umbilical artery Doppler assessment and amniotic fluid measurement), and continual/frequent assessment of fetal wellbeing by CTG. Administration of corticosteroids to accelerate fetal lung maturity in prematurity is common.

> **Box 6.5 Signs and symptoms of fulminating or worsening pre-eclampsia**
>
> - Continuing rise in blood pressure;
> - Increasing proteinuria/oliguria;
> - Development of epigastric or right upper quadrant pain/severe pain below the ribs/ liver tenderness;
> - Nausea and vomiting;
> - Cerebral disturbances (headache, altered consciousness);
> - Visual field disturbances (blindness, flashing lights, loss of visual field);
> - Papilloedema (congestion of optic disc);
> - Rapidly-progressive oedema (frequently can be easily observed on the woman's face);
> - Signs of clonus;
> - Abnormalities in fetal assessment, including reduced liquor volume and/or deterioration of CTG recording;
> - Deteriorating renal function tests;
> - Abnormal liver enzymes (ALT or AST above 70 iu/l);
> - Bleeding tendency: platelet count decreasing (below $100 \times 10^9/l$) and/or clotting factors abnormality.

Multidisciplinary team

NICE[2] suggests that discussion with neonatal paediatricians and obstetric anaethetists should take place and decisions made should be clearly documented. The most effective approach is likely to be multidisciplinary, involving obstetrician and anaesthetist at consultant level, plus haematologist, paediatrician and appropriately-experienced midwives who should all be involved in the planning and provision of care. The neonatal intensive care unit should be alerted and kept updated.

Labour/postnatal issues

If the woman's condition stabilises sufficiently to enable labour to be induced, an epidural anaesthesia is often selected if the clotting studies are satisfactory. This method of pain relief offers the additional benefits of possibly lowering blood pressure and avoids the possibility of complications that may accompany general anaesthesia and exacerbate pulmonary oedema. However, fluid management is vital for this compromised woman, and midwifery assessment of it needs to be meticulous, as is an awareness that the need for anti-hypertensive drugs may be influenced by the magnesium sulphate infusion.

Postnatal care needs to continue with the knowledge that, although delivery of the baby is deemed to be the 'cure' for pre-eclampsia, symptoms can continue or even escalate in the initial period after the birth, and therefore intensity of assessment of medications/monitoring may need to be maintained or even increased.

Complications

An awareness of potential complications (see Box 6.6) will ensure the midwife's assessment addresses these issues, and that escalation is prompt if suspicions arise.

Box 6.6 Potential maternal complications[6,19] of PET

- placental abruption;
- pulmonary oedema/aspiration;
- acute renal failure;
- liver failure or haemorrhage;

- stroke;
- long-term cardiovascular morbidity;
- visual compromise/blindness.

Eclampsia

Eclampsia is the occurrence of convulsions that are associated with the signs and symptoms of pre-eclampsia. It is a Greek word meaning 'lightning' and often strikes with the same random ferocity and has similarly devastating effects. The randomness is illustrated by the fact that 38% of seizures occur before proteinuria and hypertension have been documented.[20] The seizure that is the key feature of eclampsia is thought to be due to intense vasospasm of the cerebral arteries, oedema secondary to ischaemic damage of vascular endothelium and/or intravascular clot formation.

The occurrence of eclampsia has declined over recent years. Knight et al.[21] for UKOSS found that rates of eclampsia were down to 26.8 per 100,000 maternities, from 46 per 100,000 maternities previously. This may directly result from increasingly common use of magnesium sulphate as a treatment to prevent those with moderate/severe pre-eclampsia developing eclampsia.[22,23]

Investigations, management and ongoing assessment

Immediate care of the woman with eclampsia:

- Summon assistance (anaesthetist and obstetrician) urgently.
- Protect from injury during the tonic–clonic phase.
- Maintain airway (clear by suctioning if necessary).
- Provide supplementary oxygenation.
- Place woman in the left lateral (recovery) position.
- Obtain intravenous access and monitor fluid balance.
- Treat the convulsion (magnesium sulphate is usual).
- Monitor vital signs and beware abruption/PPH.
- Achieve stability of maternal condition.
- Assess fetal wellbeing (risk of fetal distress from hypoxia or abruption).
- If antenatal, plan mode of delivery and execute promptly.

In rare situations where seizures are recurrent or prolonged, the woman may need to be medically paralysed and ventilated. However, it is more usual for the woman to be successfully stabilised, and then receive close monitoring by the midwife, both before and after delivery. It must be remembered that, despite birth being the 'cure' for pre-eclampsia, eclampsia has been reported as occurring for the first time after delivery in many studies.[24,25] Therefore, care and careful assessment needs to continue into the postpartum period as appropriate.

Vital signs

Close attention to the assessment of respirations and BP is necessary, especially if the woman is receiving a magnesium sulphate infusion (see Box 6.7 for a list of signs and symptoms of magnesium sulphate toxicity). Magnesium sulphate is a powerful depressant of neuromuscular transmission, and care must be taken to avoid sudden hypotension, in particular if the woman is concurrently receiving large doses (especially if administered intravenously) of antihypertensives. Apart from regular and frequent monitoring of vital signs whilst receiving magnesium sulphate, the woman's deep tendon reflexes should also be monitored, usually hourly.

Continuous O_2 saturation monitoring is usual, with oxygen administration if necessary. Commencement of a cardiac monitor for ongoing ECG is common because of the potential effect on the cardiac system by magnesium sulphate.

Blood tests

PET bloods (see Box 6.4) will be sent, and repeated as necessary. A fingertip blood glucose test may be carried out. ABG may be necessary.

Regular renal function tests are usual if a woman is receiving a magnesium sulphate infusion (see 'Drugs' section in this chapter).

Fluid balance

An indwelling urinary catheter with hourly urometer to enable close monitoring of output will be used. A drop in normal urine output in a woman receiving IV magnesium sulphate will put her at risk of magnesium toxicity.

All fluid input is carefully monitored. The woman is likely to have IV magnesium sulphate and possibly IV antihypertensive medication, as well as other infusions or oral intake. Since fluid restriction is usual, careful calculation of the fluid balance is important.

Fluid restriction is likely to continue until a good urinary output is achieved.

Drugs

All maternity units will have a protocol outlining how magnesium sulphate is administered. NICE[4] suggest it is given intravenously as a loading dose of 4 g over 5 minutes, followed by a maintenance infusion of 1 g/hour for 24 hours. A seizure, or repeat seizure, should be treated with a further dose of 2–4 g given over 5 minutes. Close monitoring of women receiving IV magnesium sulphate is necessary.

A maximum blood magnesium level of 4 mmol/l is therapeutic, but around 7 mmol/l is associated with respiratory distress, while levels of around 12 mmol/l can trigger cardiac arrest. A serum magnesium level may be measured if urinary output is diminished, but it is more common to monitor renal function tests regularly while a magnesium sulphate infusion is in progress[9] to identify failing renal function, which could lead to magnesium toxicity. The midwife should be assessing for signs and symptoms of magnesium sulphate toxicity (see Box 6.7)

Box 6.7 Signs and symptoms of magnesium sulphate toxicity

- Loss of tendon reflexes
- Double vision
- Depressed respiration
- Slurred speech

- Flushing
- Weakness
- Reduced urinary output < 0.5 ml/kg/hr
- Drowsiness.

Magnesium sulphate toxicity can be treated with calcium gluconate IV, and the midwife should ensure this is easily available.

HELLP syndrome

HELLP (Haemolysis, Elevated Liver enzymes and Low Platelets) syndrome is a serious complication usually associated with pre-eclampsia but in which many women do not develop significant hypertension or proteinuria.[7,26] Diagnosis is based on a combination of laboratory findings, clinical signs and symptoms (see Box 6.8), although these may vary significantly. It has been suggested that 20% of women had not been diagnosed with pre-eclampsia before delivery and one third of women with HELLP syndrome will be diagnosed postnatally.[26] HELLP is the most common cause of severe liver disease in pregnancy.

Signs and symptoms

The most common presenting signs for those women with HELLP include epigastric or abdominal pain, nausea or vomiting, headache, visual changes, new-onset hypertension and/or new-onset proteinuria.[27] See Box 6.8 for further symptoms.

The multisystem failure in HELLP is also associated with changes in renal and hepatic function. Evidence of anaemia may indicate excessive breakdown of red cells, one of the early features of HELLP. Irrespective of the cause of anaemia (haemolysis or iron deficiency) it must be borne in mind that its presence will increase the cardiac workload and thus exacerbate hypertension. Infarctions and oedema occurring in the liver will impair its capacity to maintain adequate metabolic activities such as synthesis of clotting factors, while an increase in liver size may lead to capsular rupture triggering a combined medical, surgical and obstetric emergency. As in pre-eclampsia, thrombocytopenia develops from reduction of the life span of platelets and utilisation

---

Box 6.8 HELLP syndrome: possible signs and symptoms

- Right upper quadrant pain (and often with a positive liver recoil test)
- Epigastric pain
- Nausea and vomiting
- Malaise
- Fatigue

- Generalised oedema
- Headache
- Gastro-intestinal bleed
- Hypertension
- Proteinuria
- Reduced urine output.

---

at sites of endothelial damage. In addition, reduced circulatory volume, ischaemia, renal tubular necrosis and reduced renal clearance lead to a rise in the serum levels of urea, creatinine and urate, which are indicators of marked maternal and fetal compromise.

On admission, it can be difficult to differentiate between several conditions, especially when there is liver involvement: HELLP and AFLP symptoms can also be caused by hepatitis, thrombotic microangiopathy, thrombotic thrombocytopenic purpura, SLE, antiphospholipid syndrome and severe sepsis.[28] Women are likely to be admitted to critical care feeling very unwell, but without a definite diagnosis. The midwife is well-placed to observe signs and symptoms, as well as trends in bloods and vital signs, to aid diagnosis.

For some women, the condition may develop rapidly, while for others the progression of disease may be more gradual.

Investigations, management and ongoing assessment

Vital signs

An ABCDE check, plus a top-to-toe midwifery examination, as described for pre-eclampsia, will provide information to enable effective diagnosis, treatment and timing of delivery.

Blood tests

Possible laboratory findings:[27]

- Haemolysis (abnormal peripheral blood smear, or elevated bilirubin);
- Anaemia;
- Low platelet count ($< 100 \times 10^9$/l);
- Elevated liver enzymes:
  - Alanine aminotransferase (ALT): > 70 iu/l;
  - Gamma-glutamyltransferase (GGT): > 70 iu/l;
  - Aspartate aminotransferase (AST): > 70 iu/l.

Fluid balance

The same dangers of fluid overload in pre-eclampsia will also complicate HELLP syndrome, so fluid restriction may be necessary. An indwelling urinary catheter with an hourly urometer may be used – if not, careful measurement of all urine passed is required if accurate fluid balance is to be achieved.

Drugs

Control of blood pressure with anti-hypertensive medication if necessary, with ongoing evaluation of effectiveness of any drugs used.

Prevention of seizure (see discussion on the use of magnesium sulphate earlier in this chapter).

Fetal assessment

Assessment and monitoring of fetal condition by appropriate means: CTG, USS with Dopplers and amniotic fluid measurement.

Potential HELLP complications

Morbidity is common among women with HELLP syndrome and includes reactions to the blood products administered, admissions to intensive/critical care, eclampsia, renal impairment or failure, pulmonary oedema, subarachnoid haemorrhage, sepsis, subcapsular liver haematoma and hepatic encephalopathy. Risks to the fetus/neonate include fetal demise, IUGR, stillbirth and prematurity.[27]

1% or more of women with HELLP syndrome have a subcapsular hepatic haematoma. Hepatic haematomas can also complicate pregnancies where DIC is present.[29] Common signs and symptoms to be evaluated are in Box 6.9, but for an accurate diagnosis CT (computed tomography) scanning, ultrasound or MRI will be used. If the haematoma ruptures this is an emergency, and the woman will probably present with acute shock symptoms.[29]

Box 6.9 Potential signs and symptoms of hepatic haematoma

- Right upper quadrant, epigastric or right shoulder pain
- Pyrexia
- Hypotension
- Hepatomegaly
- Hepatic tenderness and rebound tenderness with peritonitis

- Shock, renal or respiratory failure
- Leucocytosis
- Anaemia
- Highly-elevated serum aminotransferase.

Acute fatty liver of pregnancy (AFLP)

AFLP is a rare (1:7,000 to 1:20,000) but severe condition. Although maternal mortality of 10–20% and perinatal mortality of 20–30% has been suggested,[30] in the most recent extensive UK study[31] the maternal mortality rate was 1.8% and perinatal mortality 10.4%.

The physiology of AFLP is not yet clearly identified, but it is thought that AFLP may be a variant of PET. It is characterised by hepatic microvesicular steatosis associated with mitochondrial dysfunction. It is related to an autosomal inherited mutation that causes deficiency of the long chain 3 hydroxyacyl co-enzyme A dehydrogenase (LCHAD), a fatty acid beta-oxidation enzyme.[29] Some women may be heterozygous for LCHAD deficiency (disorder of mitochondrial fatty acid oxidation), and if the fetus is homozygous for beta-fatty acid oxidation, it may be that the affected fetus is producing abnormal fatty-acid metabolites[32] and AFLP may develop.

AFLP may start antenatally (usually in the third trimester), but it may not become apparent until after the birth.[30] About half of women exhibit signs of PET.[29]

Predisposing/risk factors

Predisposing/risk factors include:[31,33,34]

* primigravidae;
* association with male fetuses (3:1);
* multiple pregnancy;
* nonsteroidal anti-inflammatory drugs;
* BMI < 20.

The vague preliminary presentation of AFLP can make it challenging to diagnose. AFLP can be confused initially with HELLP syndrome,[35] fulminant hepatitis of pregnancy,[36] other liver diseases or pancreatitis,[37] but blood tests will usually identify the correct cause. Hepatic imaging is also usually undertaken to exclude other disorders or detect hepatic haemorrhage.[29]

Signs and symptoms

Signs and symptoms usually present gradually and may be fairly non-specific initially, with women complaining of anorexia, nausea, emesis (severe vomiting in 60%), malaise, fatigue and headache. About half of women may have epigastric or RUQ pain, and about half will demonstrate signs of pre-eclampsia, although usually mild.[30] There may also be hepatic tenderness (often found when the midwife does her usual palpation before starting a CTG), but there is usually no hepatomegaly. Jaundice is a late sign, usually appearing after about 2 weeks of symptoms.

As many of these symptoms may not lead to a woman seeking advice from a midwife or doctor, the first contact the woman may have can be in response to worsening of symptoms, or a severe symptom such as coagulopathy (it is suggested 90% have DIC), which is often the presenting symptom.[32] Other serious signs and symptoms may involve various systems:

- Hepatic: ascites with abnormal LFTs, fulminant liver failure, hepatic encephalopathy;
- Renal: associated kidney injury, including lactic acidosis and raised ammonia and acute renal failure;
- Pancreas: pancreatitis, hypoglycaemia (up to 70%), which may be severe; there may also be polyuria, polydipsia and features of DIC;[32]
- Sepsis.[38]

It would be unusual for a woman with AFLP to be cared for by midwives in a critical care maternity unit setting – it would be more likely that she would be in an ICU. However, the woman may be initially admitted into a maternity critical care unit for assessment pending diagnosis, and the midwife's assessments may be critical in reaching a diagnosis as quickly as possible. This is true for all conditions, but particularly for AFLP where diagnosis is achieved by identifying signs and symptoms on a criteria list (see Box 6.10). The 'Swansea criteria for diagnosis of acute fatty liver of pregnancy' list is accepted at present for a clear diagnosis, but other markers may also be taken into consideration.[35] Liver biopsy is the gold standard diagnostic test but is rarely done due to coagulopathy.

Box 6.10 Swansea criteria for diagnosis of acute fatty liver of pregnancy[31]

Six or more criteria are required in the absence of another cause.

- Vomiting
- Abdominal pain
- Polydipsia/polyuria
- Encephalopathy
- Elevated bilirubin > 14 μmol/l
- Hypoglycaemia < 4 mmol/l
- Elevated urea > 340 μmol/l
- Leukocytosis > 11 × 10^9/l
- Ascites or bright liver on ultrasound scan

- Elevated transaminases (AAT or ALT) < 42 iu/l
- Elevated ammonia > 47 μmol/l
- Renal impairment; creatinine > 150 μmol/l
- Coagulopathy; prothrombin time > 14 seconds or APPT > 34 seconds
- Microvesicular steatosis on liver biopsy.

Investigations, management and ongoing assessment

Vital signs

Due to the uncertain diagnosis, a full range of vital signs are undertaken and repeated frequently in order to obtain a trend. Close monitoring of oxygen saturations and respirations may indicate early deterioration of the woman's condition.

Blood tests

As with vital signs, a full range of blood tests is necessary, with particular attention to liver function tests, renal function tests and clotting factors.

Blood tests may show serum aminotransferase and bilirubin levels elevated, as well as a prolonged prothrombin time, hypofibrinogenaemia and increased ammonia, uric acid, blood urea nitrogen and creatinine.

Fluid balance

A woman presenting with signs of AFLP will usually have a history of vomiting, and will need appropriate IV fluid replacement. However, as she may also have signs of polyuria and/or compromised renal function, close fluid balance is necessary in order to evaluate her condition. An indwelling urinary catheter with a urometer for hourly measurement is usual.

Potential outcome

AFLP is considered a medical and obstetrical emergency,[38] and early diagnosis and treatment will help improve survival/recovery of both the woman and fetus. Following stabilisation of the woman's condition, the baby will be delivered and, as the woman with AFLP is usually very ill, she will be cared for in a critical care or intensive care unit. In acute cases, a liver transplant may be considered.

References

1. Tranquilli, A, Dekker, G, Magee, L, Roberts, J, Sibai, BM, Zeeman, GG and Brown, MA. 2014. The classification, diagnosis and management of the hypertensive disorders of pregnancy: a revised statement from the ISSHP. *Pregnancy Hypertension*, 4(2): 97–104.
2. Nair, M and Knight, M. 2016. Maternal mortality in the UK 2012–14: surveillance and epidemiology. In: Knight, M, Nour, M, Tuffnell, D, Kenyon, S, Shakespeare, J, Brocklehurst, P and Kurinczuk, JJ (eds) on behalf of MBRRACE-UK. *Saving lives, improving mothers' care: surveillance of maternal deaths in the UK 2012–14 and lessons learned to inform maternity care from the UK and Ireland confidential enquiries into maternal deaths and morbidity 2009–14.* Oxford, UK: National Perinatal Epidemiology Unit, University of Oxford, pp. 11–32.
3. Harding, K, Redmond, P and Tuffnell, D on behalf of the MBRRACE-UK hypertensive disorders of pregnancy chapter writing group. 2016. Caring for women with hypertensive disorders of pregnancy. In: Knight, M, Nour, M, Tuffnell, D, Kenyon, S, Shakespeare, J, Brocklehurst, P and Kurinczuk, JJ (eds) on behalf of MBRRACE-UK. *Saving lives, improving mothers' care: surveillance of maternal deaths in the UK 2012–14 and lessons learned to inform maternity care from the UK and Ireland confidential enquiries into maternal deaths and morbidity 2009–14.* Oxford, UK: National Perinatal Epidemiology Unit, University of Oxford, pp. 69–75.
4. National Institute for Health and Clinical Excellence (NICE). 2010. Hypertension in pregnancy: NICE clinical guideline 107. Last modified: January 2011. Manchester, UK: NICE.
5. Bothamley, J and Boyle, M. 2009. *Medical conditions affecting pregnancy and childbirth.* Oxford, UK: Radcliffe.

6. Sibai, B, Dekker, G and Kupferminc, M. 2005. Pre-eclampsia. *Lancet*, 365(9461): 785–99.
7. Powrie, R and Rosene-Montella, K. 2008. Preeclampsia. In: Rosene-Montella, K, Keely, E, Barbour, LA and Lee, RV (eds). *Medical care of the pregnant patient*. Philadelphia, PA: ACP Press, pp. 163–81.
8. Poon, LC, and Nicolaides, KH. 2014. Early prediction of preeclampsia. *Obstetrics and Gynecology International*, 2014: 297397. Doi: 10.1155/2014/297397.
9. Higgins, L and Heazell, A. 2012. Severe preeclampsia and eclampsia. In: Chandraharan, E and Arulkumaran, S (eds). *Obstetric and intrapartum emergencies: a practical guide to management*. Cambridge, UK: Cambridge University Press, pp. 24–32.
10. Lie, R, Rasmussen, S, Brunborg, H, Gjessing, HK, Lie-Nielsen, E and Irgens, L. 1998. Fetal and maternal contributions to risk of pre-eclampsia: population based study. *British Medical Journal*, 316: 1343–7.
11. Skjaerven, R, Vatten, L, Wilcox, A, Rønning, T, Irgens, L and Lie, R. 2005. Recurrence of pre-eclampsia across generations: exploring fetal and maternal genetic components in a population based cohort. *British Medical Journal*, 331(7521): 877–85.
12. El-Moselhy, E, Khalifa, H, Amer, S, Mohammad, K and El-Aal, H. 2011. Risk factors and impacts of pre-eclampsia: an epidemiological study among pregnant mothers in Cairo, Egypt. *Journal of American Science*, 7(5): 311–23.
13. Sparks, TN, Cheng, YW, Phan, N and Caughey, AB. 2013. Does risk of preeclampsia differ by twin chorionicity? *Journal of Maternal–Fetal and Neonatal Medicine*, 26(13): 1273–7.
14. Lisonkova, S and Joseph, K. 2013. Incidence of preeclampsia: risk factors and outcomes associated with early- versus late-onset disease. *American Journal of Obstetrics and Gynecology*, 209(6): 544–6.
15. Walker, J. 2000. Severe pre-eclampsia and eclampsia. *Baillières Clinical Obstetrics and Gynaecology*, 14(1): 57–71.
16. Lewis, G (ed.). 2007. The confidential enquiry into maternal and child health (CEMACH). Saving mothers' lives: reviewing maternal deaths to make motherhood safer – 2003–2005. The seventh report on confidential enquiries into maternal deaths in the United Kingdom. London: CEMACH.
17. Côté, A, Brown, M, Lam, E, von Dadelszen, P, Firoz, T, Liston, RM and Magee, LA. 2008. Diagnostic accuracy of urinary spot protein : creatinine ratio for proteinuria in hypertensive pregnant women: systematic review. *British Medical Journal*, 335(7651): 103–6.
18. Nathan, H, Duhig, K, Hezelgrave, N, Chappell, L and Shennan, A. 2015. Blood pressure measurement in pregnancy. *The Obstetrican and Gynaecologist*, 17(2): 91–8.
19. Samra, K. 2013. The eye and visual system in the preeclampsia/eclampsia syndrome: what to expect? *Saudi J Ophthalmology*, 27(1): 51–3.
20. Magowan, B and the SCOTTIE Working Group (eds) on behalf of the Scottish Multiprofessional Maternity Development Group. 2011. Scottish core obstetric teaching and training in emergencies: 'SCOTTIE' course mI. Available at www.scottishmaternity.org. Accessed 13 February 2015.
21. Knight, M on behalf of UKOSS. 2007. Eclampsia in the United Kingdom. *British Journal of Obstetrics and Gynaecology*, 114(9): 1072–8.
22. Duley, L, Meher, S and Abalos, E. 2006. Management of pre-eclampsia. *British Medical Journal*, 332(7539): 463–8.
23. Williams, J, Mozurkewich, E, Chilimigras, J and Van de Ven, C. 2008. Critical care in obstetrics: pregnancy-specific conditions. *Best Practice and Research: Clinical Obstetrics and Gynaecology*, 22(5): 825–46.
24. Chames, MC, Livingston, JC, Ivester, TS, Barton, JR and Sibai, BM. 2002. Late postpartum eclampsia: a preventable disease? *American Journal of Obstetrics and Gynecology*, 186(6): 1174–7.

25. Ginzburg, V and Wolff, B. 2009. Headache and seizure on postpartum day 5: late postpartum eclampsia. *Canadian Medical Association Journal, 180*(4): 425–8.

26. Norwitz, E, Hsu, C and Repke, J. 2002. Acute complications of preeclampsia. *Clinical Obstetrics and Gynecology, 45*(2): 308–29.

27. Fitzpatrick, K, Hinshaw, K, Kurinczuk, J and Knight, M. 2014. Risk factors, management, and outcomes of hemolysis, elevated liver enzymes, and low platelets syndrome and elevated liver enzymes, low platelets syndrome. *Obstetrics and Gynecology, 123*(3): 618–27.

28. Pourrat, O, Coudroy, R and Pierre, F. 2015. Differentiation between severe HELLP syndrome and thrombotic microangiopathy, thrombotic thrombocytopenic purpura and other imitators. *European Journal of Obstetrics and Gynecology and Reproductive Biology, 189*: 55–8.

29. Dekker, G. 2011. Hypertension. In: James, D, Steer, P, Weiner, C and Gonik, B (eds). *High risk pregnancy*. St Louis, MO: Elsevier, pp. 599–622.

30. Cowie, P and Johnston, I. 2010. Acute fatty liver of pregnancy. *Anaesthesia tutorial of the week 191*. Available at http://e-safe-anaesthesia.org/e_library/07/Acute_fatty_liver_of_pregnancy_TOTW_191_2010.pdf.

31. Knight, M, Nelson-Piercy, C, Kurinczuk, J, Spark, P and Brocklehurst, P. 2008. A prospective national study of acute fatty liver of pregnancy in the UK. *Gut, 57*(7): 951–6.

32. Nelson-Piercy, C. 2015. *Handbook of obstetric medicine*. Boca Raton, FL: CRC Press.

33. Ko, H and Yoshida, E. 2006. Acute fatty liver of pregnancy. *Canadian Journal of Gasroenterology, 20*(1): 25–30.

34. Saygan-Karamursel, B, Kizilkilic-Parlakgumus, A, Deren, O, Onderoglue, L and Durukan, T. 2004. Care report: acute fatty liver of pregnancy. *Journal of Maternal–Fetal and Neonatal Medicine, 16*: 65–6.

35. Minakami, H, Morikawa, M, Yamada, T, Akaishi, R and Nishida, R. 2014. Differentiation of acute fatty liver of pregnancy from syndrome of hemolysis, elevated liver enzymes and low platelet counts. *Journal of Medical Ethics, 40*(3): 641–9.

36. Chen, H, Yuan, L, Tan, J, Lui, Y and Zhang, J. 2008 Severe liver disease in pregnancy. *International Journal of Gynecology and Obstetrics, 101*(3): 277–80.

37. Fesenmeier, M, Coppage, K, Lambers, D, Barton, J and Sibai, B. 2004. Acute fatty liver of pregnancy in 3 tertiary care centers. *American Journal of Obsetrics and Gynecology, 192*(5): 1416–9.

38. Schutt Vand Minuk, G. 2007. Liver diseases unique to pregnancy. *Best Practice and Research: Clinical Gastroenterology, 21*(5): 771–92.

Chapter 7

Assessment of the respiratory system

Introduction

The primary function of the respiratory system is to provide oxygen and remove carbon dioxide; consequently, a rise in respiratory rate will occur in response to illnesses in both the lungs and in other body systems (see Figure 7.1). An observation as simple as noting the respiratory rate is therefore a useful indicator of maternal health. However, assessment is complicated by a knowledge that many pregnant women experience a normal physiological sense of breathlessness, also known as shortness of breath (SOB).

The respiratory rate will rise in cases of metabolic acidosis, such as diabeticketoacidosis and sepsis, as the body tries to correct the blood pH. The respiratory rate will go up in cases of severe anaemia. When there is not enough haemoglobin, the body attempts to maintain homeostasis by increasing oxygen input through increasing respiration. Breathing will also be affected when there are problems with cardiac function, which will affect the efficiency of blood circulation. See Box 7.1 for a list of serious respiratory conditions that may affect pregnant women. The most common cause of respiratory deaths in pregnant and postpartum women in recent years has been influenza.[1]

A rise in respiratory rate will occur normally in response to exercise and can be a feature of anxiety, although caution should be applied before dismissing a raised respiratory rate as 'psychological' in cause. Women with a physical cause of increased respiratory effort will become understandingly anxious as they fight for breath. However, anxiety over-ventilation – so-called 'panic attacks' – are a very frightening experience and the midwife will need to use her skills of communication and support to help a woman control her breathing back to normal levels.

Early identification of significant changes in respiratory function is crucial to identify a woman who is becoming unwell and ensure she receives appropriate care in a timely fashion.

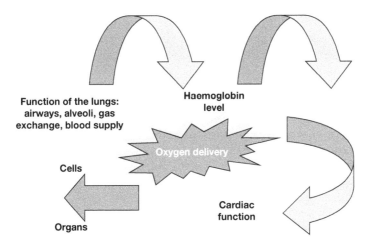

Figure 7.1 Oxygen delivery

Box 7.1 Serious respiratory conditions that may affect pregnant women

- Exacerbations of asthma;
- Respiratory infections – influenza, chicken pox, TB;
- Pneumonia – secondary to aspiration, bacterial or viral infections;
- Pulmonary embolism;
- Pulmonary oedema;
- Hyperventilation in ketoacidosis;
- Anaphylaxis;
- Cystic fibrosis;
- Acute chest syndrome in sickle cell crisis.

Physiology

Physiological adaptations to the respiratory system in pregnancy occur in response to the increased oxygen requirements of mother and fetus. These changes are driven predominantly by progesterone, which acts to increase minute ventilation. This is achieved by a 30–50% increase in tidal volume and a slight increase in respiratory rate to around 12–15 breaths per minute.[2] This enhanced maternal ventilation results in increased arterial oxygenation (pO_2) and reduced arterial carbon dioxide (pCO_2).

A benefit of this lower maternal pCO_2 is that it facilitates fetal/maternal gas exchange at the placental bed.[2] The lower maternal pCO_2 also results in a compensatory fall in serum bicarbonate. As a consequence, there is a normal, mild, fully-compensated respiratory alkalosis in pregnancy with arterial pH at around 7.44.[3] Many women become aware of this physiological increase in ventilation, noting a sense of breathlessness. The challenge for midwifery assessment is to distinguish between the normal breathlessness of pregnancy and breathlessness as a sign of deteriorating illness (see section entitled 'Assessment of breathlessness in pregnancy').

As pregnancy progresses, the uterus displaces the diaphragm upwards, decreasing functional residual capacity, although the thoracic rib cage splays out to help compensate for this.[4] This may make it more difficult for pregnant women to clear secretions, which is one of the reasons they are more at risk of pneumonia. The presence of the fetus makes emergency artificial ventilation of the lungs more difficult, and therefore, in cases of maternal cardio respiratory resuscitation, it is recommended that urgent Caesarean section is performed to enable the best chance of recovery for the mother.[5]

A further consideration of respiratory compromise in a pregnant woman is an increased risk of developing pulmonary oedema. Increased permeability of the endothelial linings of capillary blood vessels in the lungs results in fluid moving more easily into the interstitial tissue of the lungs, creating an increase in extravascular lung water. Pregnancy is also known to reduce the colloid oncotic pressure of blood and this further exacerbates the leakage of fluid from the circulation. It is much the same mechanism that results in women having oedema around their ankles, but in a more serious location. The oedema in the lung tissue results in alveolar collapse, causing a mismatch of ventilation and perfusion and the lowering of arterial oxygenation.[6] Pre–eclampsia is known to exacerbate this problem. This potential for fluid overload underpins the need for fluid restriction and careful monitoring of fluid balance in pregnant women when they are unwell.

The changes in pregnancy and vulnerability to serious complications may persist into the immediate postnatal period, and the concern applied in pregnancy will apply for at least 2 weeks postnatally.[7] See Box 7.2 for a summary of physiological changes that affect the respiratory system in pregnancy.

Box 7.2 Summary of physiological changes that affect the respiratory system in pregnancy[2,3,4,8]

- 30% ↑ in oxygen consumption due to ↑ metabolic demand for oxygen by maternal body and fetoplacental unit;
- Lower reserves of oxygen and a greater susceptibility to hypoxia;
- Position of diaphragm rises as fetus grows, impeding ventilation;
- ↑ transverse diameter of chest – this may make it more difficult to clear secretions;
- Mild respiratory alkalosis – facilitates fetal/maternal gradient gas exchange, although subjective feelings of breathlessness are common;
- Respiratory rate slightly increases to 12–15 breaths per minute at rest;
- Increased vulnerability to pulmonary oedema due to changes in oncotic pressure;
- Increased oedema of the upper airway can make intubation more difficult;
- Increased risk of infection;
- Change to coagulation increases susceptibility to pulmonary embolism;
- Need to deliver baby to effectively ventilate.

Clinical assessment of the respiratory system

Respiratory assessment will form part of an overall assessment of the woman, which will encompass ABCDE assessment (Chapter 1) alongside traditional midwifery head-to-toe examination. A systematic approach that involves the midwife assessing and documenting both subjective and objective data is advocated. This section will elaborate, with regard to specific assessment of the respiratory system, on the more common reasons women may develop problems affecting the respiratory system in pregnancy.

Assessment by the midwife

General appearance and history

Assessment normally begins with the midwife observing the woman for her general appearance, asking how she is and gathering information about the woman's relevant medical and obstetric history including current medications (see Box 7.3 for features/risk factors that would be relevant as part of assessment for respiratory illness). When listening to the woman's verbal response, the midwife is assessing her airway and breathing and will pick up on any breathlessness.

A general head-to-toe midwifery assessment will determine factors such as gestation, fetal wellbeing, bleeding or pain that will be important for identifying any causes and inform priorities for her care.

Box 7.3 Risk factors for serious respiratory illness in pregnancy

- Pre-existing conditions including asthma, diabetes, cardiac disease, anaemia, cystic fibrosis and renal disease;

- Risk factors for venous thromboembolism (VTE), such as thrombophilia, immobility, Caesarean section; swollen, painful calf indicative of deep vein thrombosis (DVT);

- Recent travel and/or contact with infectious conditions such as tuberculosis (TB), influenza and chicken pox;

- Smoking;

- Substance abuse;

- Poor nutrition;

- Obesity;

- Immune suppression including HIV.

Basic observations

Observations of respiratory rate, pulse, blood pressure, temperature and oxygen saturations should be made and recorded on the MEOWS chart. The respiratory rate should be assessed for a full minute when the woman is rested. This is best done after counting the pulse and while still holding the woman's wrist, so the midwife is able to observe the respirations without the woman being aware. When observing, the midwife will note any use of accessory muscles, such as drawing up the shoulders, and listen for any breath sounds such as wheezing (see Box 7.4 for description of breath sounds and their significance). Women whose respiratory rate has increased at rest will begin to talk in short sentences, pausing to take a breath. In response to the increased work of breathing and diminished oxygen there will be a corresponding increase in heart rate. Feelings of significant breathlessness may lead to panic, anxiety and fear. The midwife will need to try to assist the woman in deep, slow breathing, with supplemental oxygen to improve ventilation. Infection may be indicated if the temperature is raised, although the temperature can be normal or low in cases of sepsis. Box 7.5 lists some specific features the midwife may note in her assessment of respiratory function. Breathlessness (symptom), increased respiratory rate (sign), as well as reduced oxygen saturations, tachycardia and changes in blood pressure all indicate deteriorating respiratory function. Box 7.6 lists features of deteriorating respiratory function.

Box 7.4 Abnormal breath sounds that may be heard without a stethoscope[9]

- Wheezing: characteristically on expiration, as air is forced through a narrowed bronchial airway – such as occurs in asthma. The CMACE report[10] recommended that pulmonary oedema be considered as a possible cause of a 'wheeze' in a pregnant woman, especially in those not known to have asthma.

- Stridor: a croaking noise that is louder during inspiration and could indicate and obstruction of the airway.

- 'Rattly' chest: noisy breathing caused by secretions. This occurs in chest infection or more seriously in pulmonary oedema

---

Assessment of breathlessness in pregnancy

One of the challenges of assessment of the respiratory system in pregnancy is distinguishing between the physiological breathlessness experienced by many pregnant women and breathlessness (also known as shortness of breath (SOB)) of a more serious cause. Normal breathlessness comes on gradually over a number of weeks and is not associated with other adverse signs or symptoms. The woman may notice it when she is talking, although, paradoxically, it may get better with light exercise. It is more common in the third trimester but may start at any gestation.[3] However, breathlessness and an increased respiratory rate are important indications of deteriorating condition. Table 7.1 summarises potential causes of breathlessness in pregnancy, with features that will help the midwife identify serious causes of breathlessness and instigate prompt referral. The CMACE report[10] recognised 'red flag' features as useful in identifying a serious cause of breathlessness (see Box 7.7).

Box 7.5 Assessment of respiratory function by the midwife[9,11,12]

In addition to the usual set of basic observations, the midwife should observe for the following:

- Verbal response – is the woman able to complete a sentence in one breath?
- Change to the rate, depth and symmetry of breathing;
- Breath sounds – stridor, cough, wheeze?
- Skin colour – may be initially pale (vasoconstriction), but may progress to peripheral or central cyanosis;
- Decreased capillary refill;
- Signs of respiratory distress, such as sitting upright and leaning forward. Use of accessory muscles when breathing, pursed lip breathing;
- Production of sputum – blood-stained (TB, pneumonia, PE), purulent green/yellow (infection), frothy or pink (pulmonary oedema);
- Pain – chest pain with breathlessness may indicate serious cardiac problem or life-threatening PE, pleuritic pain;
- Palpitations;
- Change in level of consciousness, agitation, and confusion – may be indicative of increasing hypoxia;
- Features of acidosis, such as acetone breath noted with diabetic ketoacidosis.

Box 7.6 Features of deteriorating respiratory function[9,13]

- Increased respiratory rate: above 20 breaths per minute (time for a full minute when assessing pulse);
- Reduced respiratory rate (below 10 breaths per minute) may indicate opiate over-dose, magnesium sulphate toxicity or neurological complications;
- Breathlessness of sudden onset (see 'red flag' features in Box 7.7);
- Oxygen saturation < 95%;
- Increased supplemental oxygen required to keep oxygen saturation within normal range;
- Kussmaul breathing – deep, rapid respirations as a consequence of metabolic acidosis following diabetic ketoacidosis, sepsis, renal failure;
- CO_2 retention (as indicated by arterial blood gas (ABG) levels);
- Abnormalities of the CTG may reflect deterioration in the mother;
- Drowsiness, headache, flushed face, tremor.

Table 7.1 Possible causes of breathlessness in pregnancy[13,14]

Reason for breathlessness	Identifying features
Physiological	More common in last trimester, most apparent at rest or when speaking but paradoxically resolves during mild activity. To conclude that breathlessness is physiological, the midwife must exclude other more serious causes through careful assessment. Advise the woman that if it gets worse, or she becomes concerned about it, she should seek further assessment.
Anaemia	Breathlessness is likely only when anaemia is severe. Other more common signs of anaemia are lethargy, tiredness and dizziness. Check haemoglobin level. The midwife would note any precipitating factors such as postpartum haemorrhage.
Pulmonary embolus	Sudden onset of breathlessness associated with pleuritic or central chest pain. The woman may cough up frothy pink sputum or blood. There is an increased risk in pregnancy, but particular increased risk in the 6-week postnatal period, especially in those with risk factors (see the section on 'Thromboembolism'). A minor PE can present with features similar to a chest infection.
Cardiac causes (see Chapter 8)	Breathlessness can arise from a number of cardiac conditions. Be alert to 'red flag' features of breathlessness (Box 7.7).
Diabetic ketoacidosis (see Chapter 9)	Signs of dehydration, Kussmaul breathing (deep and laboured breathing). Ketotic breath odour.
Pneumonia	May have an associated cough, may cough up blood and may have fever. Pneumonia can occur following aspiration, or following bacterial or viral illness such as influenza and chicken pox.
Hyperventilation/anxiety	May be associated with tingling/numbing of the hands or around the mouth. Be calm and reassuring. Encourage slow breathing.
Asthma	Breathlessness with wheezing, excessive production of mucus, cough and a sensation of tightness in the chest. Symptoms are often worse at night.

Box 7.7 'Red flag' features of serious breathlessness in pregnancy[10]

- Breathlessness of sudden onset;
- Breathlessness associated with chest pain;
- Orthopnoea (difficulty breathing when lying flat) or paroxysmal nocturnal dyspnoea (a sensation of shortness of breath that wakes the woman up at night).

Advanced practitioner assessment

Chest percussion and auscultation

The doctor, midwife or nurse with advanced practitioner skills will also perform a chest examination involving percussion and auscultation. Chest percussion involves getting the woman to bend forward and cross her arms in front. This moves the scapulae laterally, giving access to the area over the lungs. The clinician places a hand on the back, over the intercostal spaces with the fingers separated, and then 'taps' with the other hand, moving down the back of the chest wall 3–4 cm at a time, repeating on both sides. The idea is to listen to the sounds from the vibrations created, to establish if the lungs are air filled, fluid filled or solid.[9] The quieter the percussion sound, the denser the medium underneath. When 'tapped' over air, the sound is loud, and over fluid, less loud; over a solid area, the sound is soft.[15] Increased resonance may occur in pneumothorax, whereas a decreased sound (dullness or flatness) over lung fields suggests alveolar collapse (atelectasis), pleural effusion or an area of cancerous growth.[16]

Auscultation involves placing a stethoscope over the right and left main bronchi, then mid lobe, then bases of lungs, to listen to breath sounds on both inspiration and expiration.[17] It will provide details of airway patency and the extent of secretions. Lung sounds can be heard clearly on the back, but, if it is difficult for the woman to sit upright, they can also be heard from the front (see Figure 7.2). When auscultating for breath sounds, make comparisons between each lung – so, listen to right then left apex, middle lobes, bases and axillae.

Sounds may be normal, abnormal, diminished or absent. Abnormal sounds include stridor (obstruction), expiratory wheeze (bronchospasm as in asthma), crackles (sputum) or pleural rub (friction between inflamed pleural surfaces).[17]

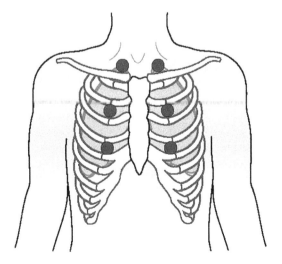

Figure 7.2 Auscultation of breath sounds: front view

Source: Philip Woodrow. 2012. *Intensive care nursing*, 3rd edition. Oxford, UK: Routledge.

Investigations

Pulse oximetry

Measurement of oxygen saturation using a probe attached to the finger, toe or ear provides a useful assessment of respiratory function. A healthy oxygen saturation reading is 95% and above. When recording the oxygen saturation, it is important to note whether the measurement is taken in room air or with supplemental oxygen. Oxygen saturation levels need to be considered in the context of assessments of pulse, BP and the level of haemoglobin and, where indicated, compared with ABG estimation.[11] Oxygen is predominantly carried by haemoglobin, and so, when haemoglobin levels are low, the blood will be delivering less total oxygen, despite normal saturation levels. Oximetry does not provide information on $PaCO_2$, and therefore ABG analysis is indicated when impairment of ventilation is noted. Box 7.8 lists factors that may affect pulse oximetry readings.

The probe should be repositioned every 4 hours and the probe site observed for complications, ensuring good blood flow and avoiding pressure damage. Check that the pulse rate recording on the saturation monitor corresponds to the woman's actual pulse.[9]

Box 7.8 Factors affecting pulse oximetry readings[11,18]

- Poor perfusion of extremities (e.g. cold limbs (vasoconstriction), oedema)
- Movement (shivering)
- Carbon monoxide (smokers)
- Dark nail varnish or false nails.

Arterial blood gases (ABG)

A test of ABG will be ordered where there is concern about deteriorating respiratory status. This will provide an assessment of levels of oxygen, carbon dioxide and any acid-base disturbance. It is assessing the effectiveness of ventilation, gaseous exchange and blood supply. Midwives will be part of a multidisciplinary team and are generally not expected to have specialist knowledge with regard to the interpretation of ABG results. However, it is useful for midwives to have a basic knowledge of the normal ranges (see Table 7.2).

A specimen of arterial blood is obtained from either the radial or femoral artery using a needle and a heparinised syringe. The woman will require a clear explanation of the test and her informed consent must be obtained. The explanation should include that it can be quite a painful procedure, and the midwife can assist the doctor taking the blood by providing support for the woman and applying pressure to the bleeding point following the procedure for at least 5 minutes, to prevent bleeding and bruising.[19] The sample taken needs to be tested quickly, within 10 minutes, although if kept in ice the time can be extended to 60 minutes. An arterial line (see Chapter 2) may be inserted to avoid the need for repeated stabs and to guide the effectiveness of treatment.[11]

Table 7.2 Normal arterial blood gas values and their significance[9,11,20]

	Normal ranges in arterial blood	Significance
pH	7.35–7.45	Acid-base balance is the maintenance of hydrogen ion (H+) balance that maintains normal cell function. Low pH: acid. High pH: alkaline. Small changes to pH outside the normal range are life threatening.
PaO_2	12.0–14.6 kPa	The partial pressure of oxygen (PO_2) dissolved in arterial blood. This indicates the amount of oxygen available for the cells.
$PaCO_2$	4.6–6.1 kPa	The partial pressure of carbon dioxide (CO_2) dissolved in arterial blood. Carbon dioxide is a waste product of cell metabolism. Increasing the respiratory rate helps the body clear carbon dioxide. This reading therefore assesses the effectiveness of ventilation.
HCO_3 (Bicarbonate)	22–26 mmol/l	Bicarbonate is an alkali. It collects hydrogen ions and neutralises them, acting as a 'buffer' or a chemical sponge for acidosis in the blood. Measurement provides a reflection of the health of the body's metabolic status.
O_2 saturation	95% and above	Oxygen is carried in the blood attached to haemoglobin molecules. Oxygen saturation is a measure of how much oxygen the blood is carrying as a percentage of the maximum it could carry.
Base excess	− 2 to + 2	Base is another word for alkali. Measurement of the surplus amount of base (alkaline) within the blood. It essentially reflects the same thing as HCO_3.

Peak flow measurement

The *peak expiratory flow rate* (PEFR) is the maximal flow (or speed) of exhalation during forced expiration, and is measured by a peak flow meter. When airways are narrowed, such as occurs in asthma, air cannot be blown out of the lungs with as much force and velocity as normal, reducing the peak flow. Results are particularly useful in measuring the woman's response to asthma medication and should be assessed after treatment.

Radiological investigations

Commonly-used radiological investigations to investigate respiratory disorders in pregnancy include chest X-ray, computed tomography of the pulmonary arteries (CTPA) and a ventilation/perfusion lung scan known as VQ scan.

Oxygen therapy

Treatment of hypoxia always involves giving oxygen therapy. It is very dry and should be humidified if used for long periods. Oxygen can be delivered by a nasal cannulae, a simple face mask (most commonly seen in a maternity unit), by a fixed performance device or via a non-rebreather mask with a reservoir bag. The latter has the benefit of achieving a higher level of oxygen by minimising room air on inspiration.[21] Continuous positive airway pressure (CPAP) is pressure that delivers oxygen into the airway by a machine, via a close-fitting mask. The advantage of CPAP is that it keeps the alveoli open at the end of expiration, improving oxygenation – although the mask is quite claustrophobic for the woman and not easily tolerated.[22] Failure to achieve oxygenation with these measures will require admission to ITU and artificial ventilation. The aim of oxygen therapy is to achieve normal oxygen saturations (95% and above).[13]

Asthma

Asthma is a chronic inflammatory disorder of the respiratory system, characterised by episodic breathlessness, wheezing, shortness of breath, excessive production of mucus, cough and a sensation of tightness in the chest. Symptoms are often worse at night. Inflammation makes the airways sensitive to stimuli, and exacerbations of asthma (asthma attacks) can be triggered by a range of factors, including infections, allergens such as pet fur and house dust mites, environmental factors such as dust and pollution, smoking and exercise. It is a preventable cause of maternal death linked to smoking and lack of education about the need to continue regular medication when pregnant.[23] It is suggested that 11–18% of pregnant women with asthma will have at least one emergency department visit for acute asthma.[24]

Severe asthma is more likely to worsen during pregnancy than mild.[24] Women with poor control of asthma in pregnancy may experience additional complications, including premature labour, pre-eclampsia and low birth weight.[23]

Investigations, management and ongoing assessment of acute severe asthma

Acute severe asthma is considered to be the triad of usual signs and symptoms of asthma but to a more serious degree: wheezing, breathlessness and a cough. Features include a respiratory rate $\geq$ 25/min, heart rate $\geq$ 110/min and an inability to complete sentences in one breath.[24] These attacks can rapidly become life-threatening, so the multidisciplinary team should be called urgently, and early transfer to intensive care is advocated.[23] In life-threatening asthma, oxygen saturation will be < 92%, the woman may be cyanosed, hypotensive, making only a weak respiratory effort and heart monitoring may show arrhythmias and/or bradycardia. She may also appear confused and finally become comatosed.[24]

Medication to control asthma and treatment for severe asthma exacerbations is the same in pregnancy as for non-pregnancy, and clinicians are advised to follow recognised guidelines.[24] Initial treatment involves high-flow oxygen therapy, with the aim to achieve oxygen saturation levels above 94%, and administration of short-acting beta agonists (SABA). The most common SABA is salbutamol, often known as Ventolin. This acts as a bronchodilator, which relaxes the muscles around the tightened airways, opening the airway. Women should have an inhaler that delivers this medication, but in a severe asthma attack the medication can be given by a nebuliser, which delivers the medication by a fine mist through a face mask, or, in severe cases, intravenously. Steroids should also be given in all cases of an acute asthma episode. Further medications may include nebulised ipratropium, magnesium sulphate, aminophylline and antibiotics if infection was the cause of the asthma attack.[3,24]

Enhanced observations of the woman, IV access, fluid balance (rehydration may be required), continuous CTG monitoring of the fetus and involvement of senior staff and the critical care team are required.[3] See Box 7.9 for recommended investigations that may help monitor ongoing assessment of acute asthma. This will be a very frightening experience for the woman: helping her to sit up, encouraging her to accept the face mask needed for oxygen therapy and nebulised medication and providing calm but focussed supportive guidance is essential.

Box 7.9 Investigations during acute severe asthma

- Continuous oxygen saturation levels.
- Arterial blood gases.
- Full blood count (FBC), urates and electrolytes (U&Es), C-reactive protein (CRP).
- Full infection screen.
- A chest X-ray may be necessary, especially if there is chest pain. There may be signs of infection, or a pneumothorax.

Influenza

Influenza is a contagious respiratory illness caused by influenza viruses. Outbreaks of influenza occur seasonally and more serious pandemic flu occurs periodically. Morbidity and mortality from influenza varies according to the viral strain, but, with all influenza, pregnant women and their newborn offspring are more vulnerable to serious complications.[25,26,27]

Although pregnant women are not more likely than non-pregnant women to contract a respiratory infection, when they do it is more likely to lead to serious complications, including pneumonia. This risk seems more pronounced in the second and third trimesters.[28] Factors such as pre-existing asthma or smoking contribute to the risk (see Box 7.10); however, problems can occur in previously-healthy women. It is considered that delays in recognition, diagnosis and treatment have contributed to many of those who have died.[29] Midwives and other healthcare providers need to educate women about the symptoms of influenza and advise them to seek medical advice if they become unwell, so that antiviral treatment (if indicated) can be started as early as possible (see Box 7.11). Ideally, this would be within 48 hours of the onset of symptoms.[30]

Box 7.10 Highest-risk categories for complications of respiratory infection in pregnancy[31]

- Smoking;
- Substance abuse;
- Poor nutrition;
- Pre-existing conditions, including asthma, diabetes, cardiac disease, anaemia and renal disease;

- Morbid obesity;
- Those with immune suppression, including human immunodeficiency virus and immunosuppressive medication.

Box 7.11 Common symptoms of influenza[32,33]

- Chills;
- Sudden onset of fever (temperature of 38 °C or above);
- Cough and sore throat;
- Generalised muscle aches and pains (especially in the back and legs);

- Severe headache;
- Weakness or fatigue;
- Loss of appetite;
- Gastrointestinal symptoms: nausea, vomiting, diarrhoea and abdominal pain.

Investigations, management and ongoing assessment of influenza

Complications of influenza for the mother include pneumonia, sepsis, haematological disorders, pneumothorax, cardiac arrhythmias, renal failure and encephalopathy.[31,34,35] Box 7.12 lists features that would indicate the development of complications for a woman with influenza. The midwife should seek urgent medical referral if these are identified on assessment. A very high or sustained maternal temperature during pregnancy has been associated with an increased risk of birth defects, including neural tube defects,[36] and for this reason the midwife should advise measures to help women keep their temperature down.

Box 7.12 Influenza – indications of deteriorating condition[37,38]

- Signs of respiratory distress – dyspnoea, tachypnoea;
- Peripheral O_2 saturation ß 94% in air;
- Pain or pressure in chest or abdomen;
- Altered conscious level, sudden dizziness, confusion or seizures;
- Dehydration, shock or any signs of sepsis;
- Severe or long-lasting vomiting;
- Bloodstained sputum;
- Decreased fetal movements;
- High temperature not controlled by paracetamol.

Table 7.3 Recommendations for the assessment and management of a woman with influenza [37,38]

Where	Admission to hospital if condition deteriorating (Box 7.12). Admission to a single room with respiratory isolation. Intensive care unit admission will be indicated if there are signs of respiratory distress, pneumonia, persistent tachycardia (> 100 beats per minute) or altered level of consciousness.
Multidisciplinary team	Consultant level obstetrician, respiratory physician, obstetric anaesthetist, midwife, haematologist, the intensive care team, infectious disease specialist and the infection prevention and control team.
Assessment by medical team	Multidisciplinary assessment for exclusion of other complications such as disseminated intravascular coagulation or obstetric complications including pre-eclampsia, chorioamnionitis, urinary tract infection and pulmonary embolism. Careful fluid monitoring and assessment required. Multidisciplinary decision needed regarding timing and mode of delivery. Preterm delivery may be indicated to improve ventilation of a very ill mother.
Midwifery observations	ABCDE assessment and regular observations including oxygen saturations; record on MEOWS chart to facilitate identification of women whose condition is deteriorating. Tachycardia and hypoxia have been noted to be clear signs of severe disease.[10] Monitor usual signs of maternal and fetal wellbeing. Midwifery head-to-toe assessment. Monitor fluid balance, including hourly urine output. Observe for signs of labour. Provide psychological support to the woman and her family. Notify infection prevention and control team and observe strict isolation and infection control measures.
Investigations	Perform appropriate bacteriological investigations including blood and sputum cultures. Blood tests as indicated. Monitor arterial blood gas. Perform chest X-ray.
Medication	Control maternal pyrexia to prevent complications including fetal abnormality and preterm delivery. Possibly use antiviral medication. Corticosteroids to promote fetal lung maturity may be used with caution. Specialist guidance should be sought. Assessment required by the medical team regarding the need for antibiotics.

Pneumonia

Pneumonia is an inflammation of the lungs caused by microorganisms, usually bacteria or viruses. The inflammation produces fluid and the small air sacs (alveoli) of the lungs become filled with fluid exudate, impairing gaseous exchange. The affected area can be confined to one portion of the lungs (lobar pneumonia) or it can be more widespread (bronchopneumonia).[11] Pneumonia accounts for nearly 20% of admissions to ITU of women who are currently pregnant.[39] The physiological changes in pregnancy make it more likely for pregnant women to have pneumonia, and, if they do, the treatment is more challenging.

Clinical features of pneumonia

The classic features of pneumonia include a dry cough, breathlessness and chest pain. There may also be fever, agitation and confusion.[40] Ventilation and perfusion are likely to be compromised, resulting in reduced O_2 saturation. An examination of the chest may note that lung expansion is reduced on the affected side. Percussion will note dullness over the consolidated area and bronchial breathing may be heard. There may be production of purulent or 'rusty' sputum as the pneumonia clears.[11]

Investigations, management and ongoing assessment of pneumonia

Blood cultures should be taken and a chest X-ray will confirm diagnosis.[41] There may be a delay in the diagnosis of pneumonia in pregnancy and this may contribute to increased morbidity. The normal breathlessness of pregnancy may mask developing disease. A distinction between these normal findings and disease can be made by detailed assessment and a chest X-ray as indicated.

The woman may be cared for in a high dependency maternity care setting, but, if her condition is poor or deteriorating and/or she requires ventilation, she is likely to be transferred into an intensive care unit.[42] Delivery of the fetus will be considered to improve ventilation of the mother.

When the woman is being cared for in a maternity setting, the midwifery responsibilities will include basic observations and respiratory assessment, positioning, O_2 therapy, monitoring fluid balance, fetal assessment, administration of medication, effective infection control measures and psychological care. When a woman is experiencing difficulty in breathing, it will help to maximise ventilation by encouraging her to adopt a high side-lying position.[13] This promotes aeration and perfusion of any healthy lung tissue.[11] This position also avoids any aortocaval compression by the uterus, which would be detrimental to mother and fetus. There should be continuous CTG monitoring as indicated. Blood flow and oxygenation to the placenta is entirely dependent on the mother's haemodynamic state, and thus fetal wellbeing requires effective treatment of the mother.[40]

O_2 therapy is recommended when there is evidence of hypoxaemia, with the aim of maintaining O_2 saturation levels at or above 95%. In cases of severe hypoxaemia, high-concentration O_2 (15 l per minute) via a non-rebreathing reservoir mask should be commenced. For those with milder hypoxaemia, O_2 can be administered via nasal cannulae at 2–6 l per minute or via a simple face mask at 5–10 l per minute.[13] Humidification is not usually necessary for low-flow O_2 therapy, but may be required when using O_2 for longer than 24 hours.[11]

Fluid replacement may be indicated. An increase in insensible water loss associated with an increased respiratory rate and fever may lead to dehydration, which can cause secretions to become stickier. Regular sips of water where possible is advocated. A fluid balance chart should be used.[11]

Pulmonary embolism

Venous thromboembolism (VTE) is the leading cause of direct maternal deaths in the UK.[43] Pulmonary embolism (PE) is the most common cause of death associated with

VTE. It occurs when a clot from a deep vein (DVT), commonly in the leg, detaches itself and travels to the lungs, where it lodges in a pulmonary blood vessel. Collapse and death will occur if the clot is large enough to compromise the pulmonary circulation. Therefore, recognition and treatment of DVT is important in limiting deaths from PE.

Pregnancy combines features of hypercoagulability, venous stasis and vascular damage, making pregnant and postnatal women more prone to VTE.

Risk assessment for VTE

Computer-generated and paper-based risk assessment tools that aim to identify women at higher risk of VTE have been in common use for the last decade.[44] These have enabled timely thromboprophylaxis, which aims to prevent VTE, including anticoagulant medication (usually low molecular weight heparin: LMWH) and thromboembolic deterrent stockings (TEDS). An assessment for risk factors for VTE should be made at booking, repeated if admitted to hospital, or if factors change, and again immediately postpartum. For any woman presenting with features of pulmonary embolism, a review of risk factors (Box 7.13) and evidence of deep vein thromboses (Box 7.14) would contribute to the diagnosis of PE.

Box 7.13 Risk factors for VTE in pregnancy and the postpartum period[44,45,46,47]

General factors:

- Personal or family history of DVT, PE or thrombophilia;
- Age over 35;
- Obesity (BMI > 30);
- Prolonged immobilisation; e.g., paraplegia, air travel;
- Major current illness; e.g., malignancy, diabetes and/or heart, lung, kidney or bowel disease;
- Mechanical heart valves;
- Sickle-cell disease;
- Major varicose veins;
- Smoking.

Pregnancy-related factors:

- Caesarean section;
- Parity ≥ three;
- Multiple pregnancy;
- Assisted reproduction. Ovarian hyperstimulation syndrome (OHSS);
- Severe infection;
- Pre-eclampsia;
- Stillbirth;
- Preterm birth;
- Immobility (including bed rest, symphysis pubis dysfunction);
- Surgical procedures in pregnancy;
- Prolonged labour, instrumental delivery;
- Dehydration, hyperemesis;
- Excessive blood loss.

Box 7.14 Symptoms and signs of DVT[48,49,50]

- Pain in calf, thigh, groin, buttocks (especially unilateral pain);
- Swelling (at least 3 cm difference between the two legs when measured 10 cm below the tibial tuberosity);
- Redness or discolouration or change in temperature of the affected leg;
- Homan's sign (pain on dorsiflexion of the foot) (unreliable);
- Low-grade pyrexia (37.5 °C);
- Tachycardia (pulse > 100/min);
- Lower abdominal pain;
- Limb symptoms on left side (> 80%).[47]

Assessment of clinical signs of pulmonary embolism

The clinical signs of PE (see Box 7.15) are related to the size of the clot that is obstructing the pulmonary circulation. Large or multiple emboli will prevent adequate oxygenation of the blood. A woman with a major PE will collapse with severe breathlessness, cyanosis, hypotension and chest pain. Sudden respiratory or cardiac arrest may occur. Warning signs and symptoms indicative of smaller emboli include unexplained pyrexia, cough, chest pain and breathlessness, which may be incorrectly diagnosed as a chest infection or be explained away as normal breathlessness of pregnancy. Midwives need to identify all possible pulmonary embolism symptoms so

---

Box 7.15 Clinical manifestations of PE[48,49]

Most frequent signs and symptoms:

- Sudden or unexpected difficulty in breathing;
- Increased respiratory rate;
- Feeling faint;
- Tightness in chest or pleuritic chest pain;

- Increased pulse;
- Cough;
- Crackles on lung auscultation;
- DVT.

Associated signs and symptoms:

- Coughing up blood;
- Distended neck veins;
- Cyanosis and collapse;

- Hypotension;
- Anxiety;
- Low-grade fever.

Assessed in combination with signs and symptoms of DVT.

---

that prompt referral, pursuit of an accurate diagnosis and initiation of effective treatment can be made. Failure to identify the subtler symptoms of a PE, especially in the presence of additional risk factors, has been identified as a contributing factor in some maternal deaths.[10]

Investigations

Compression duplex ultrasound of both limbs will normally be the initial investigation in women suspected of having a PE who also have leg symptoms. The diagnosis of DVT will indirectly confirm the diagnosis of PE, and treatment (which is the same for both conditions) can be maintained.[51]

Chest X-ray. A chest X-ray will identify other causes for chest symptoms, such as pneumonia, as well as show changes that may be indicative of PE. The radiation dose from a chest X-ray is considered negligible.[52]

A *ventilation/perfusion* (V/Q) *scan* consists initially of assessment of the pulmonary blood flow (perfusion), following an intravenous injection of a radioactive marker. Areas with reduced or absent perfusion are diagnostic of PE. The ventilation component of the V/Q scan collects information regarding the distribution of inhaled gas. This component may be omitted in pregnancy to reduce radiation exposure to the fetus.[51]

A *computed tomography pulmonary angiogram* (CTPA) can be used, in which the pulmonary arteries are assessed, following the injection of a dye into the blood-stream.[51]

V/Q and CTPA involve radiation exposure to mother and fetus. Agreed protocols for testing will help keep exposure to a minimum while still attaining accurate diagnosis.[51]

Laboratory tests, involving full blood count (FBC), coagulation tests, urea and electrolytes, and liver function tests.

Further assessments of the woman's condition will be undertaken with a full set of basic observations, including oxygen saturation monitoring. An *electrocardiogram* (ECG) and an *echocardiogram* (ECHO) may also be ordered to investigate PE and will also identify any cardiac causes for the woman's symptoms.[51]

Management and ongoing assessment of pulmonary embolism

As in any emergency situation, if a woman collapses with a major PE, the midwife must summon senior medical staff and implement appropriate resuscitation procedures immediately. Box 7.16 summarises the key responsibilities of the midwife when a woman is suspected of having a PE.

Sickle cell disease (acute chest syndrome)

Sickle cell disease (SCD) is a general name for a disorder where the person has inherited two unusual haemoglobin alleles, one of which is sickle haemoglobin. See Box 7.17 for some of these more common disorders. Sickle cell trait (HbAS) is the carrier state, and is a cause of mild anaemia in pregnancy. It is not considered SCD because it doesn't cause complications, although there is a one-in-four risk of major haemoglobinopathy in the fetus if both parents are carriers.

Box 7.16 Midwife's responsibilities in pulmonary embolism emergency

For women presenting with cardiovascular collapse:

- Assess airway, breathing, circulation (ABC assessment).
- Summon the emergency response team.
- Administer cardiopulmonary resuscitation (CPR) as required.
- Assist with endotracheal intubation as necessary.

And for all women suspected of having PE:

- Admit to hospital and refer to senior obstetrician, anaesthetist or physician.
- Give heparin and other drugs according to medical orders.
- Monitor oxygen saturations with pulse oximeter.
- Give oxygen via a face mask if O_2 saturations are below 95% in air. If appropriate, sit the woman up to maximise the respiratory effort.
- Record ECG.
- Initiate IV access.
- Take blood for FBC, coagulation screen, urea, electrolytes and liver function tests.
- Assess and record cardiovascular and respiratory vital signs.
- Maintain accurate fluid balance.
- Assess for bleeding.
- Monitor fetal wellbeing as appropriate.
- Support the woman and her family.

Box 7.17 Some of the more common disorders grouped under the name 'sickle cell disease'[53]

- HbSS: Sickle cell anaemia. This is the most common of the sickle cell disorders.
- HbSC: Haemoglobin SC disease.
- HbSβ thal: Sickle beta thalassaemia.

Complications of sickle cell disease

When a person with sickle cell disease experiences events such as dehydration, infection, low oxygen supply or emotional stress, their fragile red blood cells may form crystals and assume the characteristic pointed and elongated sickle shape. This causes a breakdown of RBCs and increased viscosity of the blood (predisposing to VTE), and can lead to a sickling crisis.[54] Up to 50% of women with SCD will experience a painful sickle crisis in pregnancy.[55] *Sickle cell crisis* is defined as an acute onset of severe pain, and requires medical attention. It is a broad term used to describe a group of acute events that occur in response to triggers (see Box 7.18), but the most common is the *vaso-occlusive crisis.* The abnormal cells clump and block blood from getting through capillaries. The lack of oxygen and subsequent ischaemia is very painful. The decreased amount of oxygen in the blood damages local tissues and will cause permanent damage if it lasts long enough. This may occur at any time, and pregnancy, labour and the puerperium all have great potential to precipitate a crisis.[53] Previous crises may have left residual organ or system damage, which may also compromise the woman's condition. Acute chest syndrome (ACS) is a life-threatening respiratory complication that may occur in pregnancy.[55] See Box 7.19 for complications of sickle cell disease and Table 7.4 for assessment and management of acute painful crisis in pregnancy.

Box 7.18 Triggers to sickling crises in pregnancy and childbirth

- Infection;
- Sudden change in temperature – cold or hot;
- Dehydration – related to nausea and vomiting in early pregnancy, labour;
- Physical exertion;
- Hypoxia/acidosis – related to illness and anaemia;
- Psychological stress;
- Unknown.

Box 7.19 Complications of sickle cell disease[54,56]

Long term (women may have these prior to pregnancy, and assessment in the preconception period is advised):

- Chronic anaemia;
- Damage to the spleen, increasing vulnerability to infection;
- Gallstone formation;
- Joint damage;
- Renal, liver, cardiac and respiratory disorders;
- Cerebrovascular accidents (stroke).

Pregnancy-related:

- Increased risk of vascular complications including increased sickling crisis;
- Urinary tract infection;
- Acute chest syndrome;
- Blood transfusion;
- Higher incidence of placental abruption and placenta praevia;
- Higher incidence of hypertension and pre-eclampsia;
- Higher incidence of venous thromboembolism;
- Maternal anaemia leading to fetal/newborn anaemia;
- Hypo-perfusion of the placental circulation as a result of sickling in the uterine placental decidua leading to fetal hypoxia;
- IUGR;
- Preterm and operative delivery more likely.

Table 7.4 Assessment and management of acute painful crisis in pregnancy[55,57]

Location	Women with SCD who become unwell need to be admitted to hospital urgently and be assessed for sickle cell crisis. Women receiving parental opiates should be cared for where regular observation and assessment can be made.
	May need critical/ICU care.
Multidisciplinary team	Multidisciplinary assessment will include a haematologist, an obstetrician, an anaesthetist, midwives and a sickle cell specialist nurse.
Pain relief	Pain relief should be administered rapidly. Initial analgesia should be given within 30 minutes of arriving in hospital and effective analgesia should be achieved within 1 hour.
	Opioids may be required.
Fluids	Fluid intake of at least 60 ml/kg/24 hours is recommended. There is a risk of overload if she also has PET. Senior clinicians should be involved in managing fluid balance.
Oxygen	Oxygen should be prescribed if oxygen saturations fall below 95%. Transfer the woman to ITU if not maintaining oxygenation.
Observations	Observations of BP, oxygen saturations, pulse rate, respiratory rate and temperature on admission.
	Assessments of pain severity, respiratory rate, oxygen saturations and sedation should be made at regular, frequent intervals and recorded on a MEOWS chart until pain is controlled and observations are stable. The minimum monitoring will be every 2–4 hours, which should be continued hourly if receiving parental opiates.
Examination and assessment	Assessments should be made for ACS, sepsis and dehydration. Examination should focus on the site of pain and identifying any precipitating factors (such as infection).
History	It is important to ask the woman if the pain is typical or not for her and if she is aware of any triggers. If pain is not typical, other causes should be investigated.
Medications (in addition to pain relief)	Thromboprophylaxis should be given.
	Laxative (prevent constipation), antiemetic (to treat opiate-induced sickness) and antihistamine (to treat opiate-induced itching).
	Antibiotics to treat any infection identified.
Investigations	FBC, reticulocyte count and renal function, blood cultures, liver function tests, CRP.
	Chest X-ray.
	Urine culture.
	As indicated: arterial blood gases, USS, investigations for neurological impairment.
Reduction in triggers	Maintenance of a comfortable, warm temperature and stress-free environment, as far as possible.
	Respectful, woman-centred care.
	Ensuring adequate hydration.

continued

Table 7.4 continued

Monitoring fetal wellbeing	CTG monitoring – when appropriate.
	Transient reduction in fetal movements and a reduced baseline variability of the fetal heart rate trace may be noted after administration of opiates.
	If the woman is in her third trimester, delivery may be needed to resolve complications.

Assessment and management of Acute Chest Syndrome (ACS)

Acute chest syndrome is a serious and often fatal complication due to sickling with vaso-occlusion in the lungs. Maternity staff should be aware of the possibility of acute chest syndrome in women who present with a sickle cell crisis if any of the following are noted:

- abnormal respiratory signs and/or symptoms;
- chest pain;
- fever;
- signs and symptoms of hypoxia (oxygen saturations less than 95%);[57]
- changes on the CTG.

Acute chest syndrome can complicate 7–20% of pregnancies.[55] ACS may be caused by a number of factors, including infection. Women should be closely monitored for deterioration, which may include reduced oxygen saturations, increasing respiratory rate, decreasing platelet count, decreasing haemoglobin concentration and neurological complications. Women with ACS should be given prompt and adequate pain relief. The critical care team should be consulted early for respiratory support, with admission to intensive care unit likely.[58] Treatment is challenging and may include mechanical ventilation, exchange blood transfusion, heparin and antibiotics.

Further reading

British Thoracic Society (BTS)/Scottish intercollegiate guidelines network (SIGN). 2016. SIGN 153, British guideline on the management of asthma. Available at www.brit-thoracic. org.uk/document-library/clinical-information/asthma/btssign-asthma-guideline-2016/. Accessed 12 September 2017.

National Institute for Health and Clinical Excellence (NICE). 2012. Sickle cell acute painful episode: management of an acute painful sickle cell episode in hospital. NICE clinical guideline 143. Available at www.nice.org.uk/guidance/cg143/evidence/full-guideline-pdf-186634333. Accessed 12 September 2017.

Royal College of Obstetricians and Gynaecologists (RCOG). 2015a. Green-top guideline no. 37b: thromboembolic disease in pregnancy and the puerperium: acute management. London: RCOG.

References

1. Churchill, D, Rodger, A, Clift, J and Tuffnell, D on behalf of the MBRRACE-UK sepsis chapter writing group. 2016. Think sepsis. In: Knight, M, Nour, M, Tuffnell, D, Kenyon,

S, Shakespeare, J, Brocklehurst, P and Kurinczuk, JJ (eds) on behalf of MBRRACE-UK. *Saving lives, improving mothers' care: surveillance of maternal deaths in the UK 2012–14 and lessons learned to inform maternity care from the UK and Ireland confidential enquiries into maternal deaths and morbidity 2009–14*. Oxford, UK: National Perinatal Epidemiology Unit, University of Oxford, pp. 27–45.

2. Tan, EK and Tan, EL. 2013. Alterations in physiology and anatomy during pregnancy. *Best Practice and Research: Clinical Obstetrics and Gynaecology*, 27(6): 791–802.

3. Nelson-Piercy, C. 2015. *Handbook of obstetric medicine*. Boca Raton, FL: CRC Press.

4. Annamraju, H and Mackillop, L. 2017. Respiratory disease in pregnancy. *Obstetrics, Gynaecology and Reproductive Medicine*, 27(4): 105–11.

5. Resuscitation Council UK. 2015. Pre-hospital resuscitation. Available at www.resus.org.uk/resuscitation-guidelines/prehospital-resuscitation/#changes. Accessed 1 October 2017.

6. Clutton-Brock, T. 2011. Critical care. Saving mothers' lives: reviewing maternal deaths to make motherhood safer: 2006–2008. The eighth report of the confidential enquiries into maternal deaths in the United Kingdom. *British Journal of Obstetrics and Gynaecology*, 118(1): s173–80.

7. Ramussen, SA, Kissin, DM, Yeung, LF, McFarlane, K, Chu, SY, Turcios-Ruiz, RM ... and Jamieson, DJ. 2011. Preparing for influenza after 2009 H1N1: special considerations for pregnant women and newborns. *American Journal of Obstetrics and Gynecology*, 204(6): 13–20.

8. Blackburn, ST. 2013. *Maternal, fetal and neonatal physiology*. Philadelphia: Saunders Elsevier.

9. Jevon, P and Ewens, B. 2012. *Monitoring the critically ill patient*. Oxford, UK: Wiley-Blackwell.

10. Centre for Maternal and Child Enquiries (CMACE). 2011. Saving mothers' lives: reviewing maternal deaths to make motherhood safer: 2006–2008. The eighth report of the confidential enquiries into maternal deaths in the United Kingdom. *British Journal of Obstetrics and Gynaecology*, 118(1): s1–203.

11. Margereson, C and Withey, S. 2012. The patient with acute respiratory problems. In: Peate, I and Dutton, H (eds). *Acute nursing care: recognising and responding to medical emergencies*. London: Pearson, pp. 81–106.

12. Hunter, J and Rawlings-Anderson, K. 2008. Respiratory assessment. *Nursing Standard*, 22(41): 41–3.

13. O'Driscoll, BR, Howard, L, Earis, J, Mak, V, Bajwah, S, Beasley, R ... and Wijesinghe, M. 2017. British Thoracic Society guidelines for oxygen use in adults in healthcare and emergency settings. *Thorax*, 72(1): Si1–i90.

14. Paterson-Brown, S and Howell, C (eds). 2016. *The MOET course manual: managing obstetric emergencies and trauma*. Cambridge, UK: Cambridge University Press.

15. Cox, C and McGrath, A. 1999. Respiratory assessment in critical care units. *Intensive and Critical Care Nursing*, 15(4): 226–34.

16. Albarran, J and Tagney, J. 2007. *Chest pain: advanced assessment and management skills*. Oxford, UK: Blackwell Publishing.

17. Woodrow, P. 2012. *Intensive care nursing: a framework for practice*. London: Routledge.

18. Booker, R. 2008. Pulse oximetry. *Nursing Standard*, 22(30): 39–41.

19. Hennessey, I and Japp, A. 2007. *Arterial blood gases made easy*. London: Elsevier.

20. Woodrow, P. 2016. *Nursing acutely ill adults*. London: Routledge.

21. Field, D. 2005. Respiratory care. In: Sheppard, M and Wright, M (eds). *Principles and practice of high dependency nursing*. Edinburgh, UK: Elsevier, pp. 75–106.

22. Vaughan, D, Robinson, N, Lucas, N and Arulkumaran, S. 2010. *Handbook of obstetric high dependency care*. Oxford, UK: Blackwell Publishing.

23. Nelson-Piercy, C, MacKillop, L, Williamson, C, and Griffiths, M on behalf of the MBRRACE-UK medical complications writing group. 2014. Caring for women with other medical complications. In: Knight, M, Kenyon, S, Brocklehurst, P, Neilson, J, Shakespeare, J and Kurinczuk, JJ (eds) on behalf of MBRRACE-UK. *Saving lives, improving mothers' care: lessons learned to inform future maternity care from the UK and Ireland confidential enquiries into maternal deaths and morbidity 2009–12.* Oxford, UK: National Perinatal Epidemiology Unit, University of Oxford, pp. 81–7.

24. British Thoracic Society (BTS)/Scottish Intercollegiate Guidelines Network (SIGN). 2016. SIGN 153, British guideline on the management of asthma. Available at www.britthoracic.org.uk/document-library/clinical-information/asthma/btssign-asthma-guideline-2016/. Accessed 12 September 2017.

25. Dodds, L, McNeil, SA, Fell, DB, Allen, VM, Coombs, A, Scott, J and MacDonald, N. 2007. Impact of influenza exposure on rates of hospital admissions and physician visits because of respiratory illness among pregnant women. *CMAJ, 176*(4): 463–8.

26. Jamieson, DJ, Honein, MA, Rasmussen, SA, Williams, JL, Swerdlow, DL, Biggerstaff, MS . . . and Olsen, SJ. 2009. H1N1 2009 influenza virus infection during pregnancy in the USA. *Lancet, 374*(9688): 451–8.

27. Mosby, LG, Rasmussen, SA, Jamieson, DJ. 2011. 2009 pandemic influenza A (H1N1) in pregnancy: a systematic review of the literature. *American Journal of Obstetrics and Gynecology, 205*(1): 10–18.

28. Louie, JK, Acosta, M, Jamieson, DJ, and Honein, MA. 2010. Severe 2009 H1N1 influenza in pregnant and postpartum women in California. *New England Journal of Medicine, 362*(1): 27–35.

29. Knight, M, Kenyon, S, Brocklehurst, P, Neilson, J, Shakespeare, J and Kurinczuk, JJ (eds) on behalf of MBRRACE-UK. 2014. *Saving lives, improving mothers' care: lessons learned to inform future maternity care from the UK and Ireland confidential enquiries into maternal deaths and morbidity 2009–2012.* Oxford, UK: National Perinatal Epidemiology Unit, University of Oxford, pp. 57–63.

30. Ramussen, SA, Kissin, DM, Yeung, LF, McFarlane, K, Chu, SY, Turcios-Ruiz, RM . . . and Jamieson, DJ. 2011. Preparing for influenza after 2009 H1N1: special considerations for pregnant women and newborns. *American Journal of Obstetrics and Gynecology, 204*(6): 13–20.

31. Lim, BH and Mahmood, TA. 2010. Pandemic H1N1 2009 (swine flu) and pregnancy. *Obstetrics, Gynaecology and Reproductive Medicine, 20*(4): 101–6.

32. Department of Health (DH). 2013. Influenza. In: Immunisation against infectious disease: the green book [online]. Available at www.gov.uk/government/uploads/system/uploads/attachment_data/file/239268/Green_Book_Chapter_19_v5_2_final.pdf. Accessed 1 October 2017.

33. Panda, B, Panda, A and Riley, LE. 2010. Selected viral infections in pregnancy. *Obstetrics and Gynecology Clinics of North America, 37*(2): 321–31.

34. Ellington, SR, Hartman, LK, Acosta, M, Martinez-Romo, M, Rubinson, L, Jamieson, DJ and Louie, J. 2011. Pandemic 2009 influenza A (H1N1) in 71 critically ill women in California. *American Journal of Obstetrics and Gynecology, 204*(6): 21–9.

35. Pratt, R. 2009. The global swine flu pandemic 1: exploring the background to influenza viruses. *Nursing Times, 105*(34): 18–21.

36. Moretti, ME, Bar-Oz, B, Fried, S and Koren, G. 2005. Maternal hyperthermia and the risk for neural tube defects in offspring: systematic review and meta-analysis. *Epidemiology, 16*(2): 216–19.

37. Modder, J. 2010. Review of maternal deaths in the United Kingdom related to A/H1N1 2009 influenza [online]. Available at www.hqip.org.uk/assets/NCAPOP-Library/CMACE-

Reports/12.-December-2010-Review-of-Maternal-Deaths-in-the-United-Kingdom-related-to-AH1N1–2009-Influenza3.pdf. Accessed 1 October 2017.

38. Department of Health (DH), Royal College of Obstetricians and Gynaecologists (RCOG). 2009. Pandemic H1N1 2009 influenza: clinical management guidelines for pregnancy. Updated 10 December 2009; now archived. Available at http://webarchive.nationalarchives.gov.uk/20130107105354/http://www.dh.gov.uk/prod_consum_dh/groups/dh_digitalassets/@dh/@en/documents/digitalasset/dh_107840.pdf. Accessed 1 October 2017.

39. Intensive Care and National Audit Research Centre (ICNARC). 2009. Female admissions (aged 16–50 years) to adult, general critical care units in England, Wales and Northern Ireland, reported as 'currently pregnant' or 'recently pregnant': 1 January 2007 to 31 December 2007. Available at www.oaa-anaes.ac.uk/assets/_managed/editor/File/Reports/ICNARC_obs_report_Oct2009.pdf. Accessed 1 October 2017.

40. Goodnight, WH and Soper, DE. 2005. Pneumonia in pregnancy. *Critical Care Medicine*, *33*(10): S390–7.

41. Stone, S and Nelson-Piercy, C. 2012. Respiratory disease in pregnancy. *Obstetrics, Gynaecology and Reproductive Medicine*, 22(10): 290–8.

42. Paruk, F. 2008. Infection in obstetric critical care. *Best Practice and Research: Clinical Obstetrics and Gynaecology*, 22(5): 865–83.

43. Nair, M and Knight, M on behalf of the MBRRACE-UK. Maternal mortality in the UK 2012–2014: Surveillance and Epidemiology. 2016. In: Knight, M, Nair, M, Tuffnell, D, Kenyon, S, Shakespeare, J, Brocklehurst, P and Kurinczuk, JJ (eds) on behalf of MBRRACE-UK. *Saving lives, improving mothers' care: surveillance of maternal deaths in the UK 2012–2014 and lessons learned to inform maternity care from the UK and Ireland confidential enquiries into maternal deaths and morbidity 2009–2014*. Oxford, UK: National Perinatal Epidemiology Unit, University of Oxford, pp. 69–75.

44. Royal College of Obstetricians and Gynaecologists (RCOG). 2015b. Green-top guideline no. 37a: reducing the risk of venous thromboembolism during pregnancy and the puerperium. London: RCOG.

45. Jacobsen, AF, Skjeldestad, FE and Sandset, PM. 2008. Incidence and risk patterns of venous thromboembolism in pregnancy and puerperium: a register-based case-control study. *American Journal of Obstetrics and Gynecology*, *198*(2): 234.e1–e7.

46. Knight, M on behalf of UK Obstetric Surveillance System (UKOSS). 2008. Antenatal pulmonary embolism: risk factors, management and outcomes. *British Journal of Obstetrics and Gynaecology*, *115*: 453–61.

47. McClintock, C. 2014. Thromboembolism in pregnancy: challenges and controversies in the prevention of pregnancy-associated venous thromboembolism and management of anticoagulation in women with prosthetic heart valves. *Best Practice and Research: Clinical Obstetrics and Gynaecology*, 28(4): 519–36.

48. Rodger, M, Rosene-Montella, K and Barbour, L. 2008. Acute thromboembolic disease. In: Rosene-Montella, K, Keely, E, Barbour L and Lee, R (eds). *Medical care of the pregnant patient*. Philadelphia, PA: ACP Press, pp. 426–44.

49. Farquharson, RG and Greaves, M. 2011. Thromboembolic disease. In: James, DK (ed.). *High risk pregnancy: management options*. Philadelphia, PA: Saunders Elsevier, pp. 753–62.

50. *British Medical Journal*. 2016. Deep vein thrombosis. Available at http://bestpractice.bmj.com/best-practice/monograph/70/diagnosis/step-by-step.html. Accessed 29 September 2017.

51. Royal College of Obstetricians and Gynaecologists (RCOG). 2015a. Green-top guideline no. 37b: thromboembolic disease in pregnancy and the puerperium: acute management. London: RCOG.

52. Donnelly, JC and D'Alton, ME. 2013. Pulmonary embolus in pregnancy. *Seminars in Perinatology*, 37(4): 225–33.

53. Bothamley, J and Boyle, M. 2009. Medical conditions affecting pregnancy and childbirth. Oxford, UK: Radcliffe.
54. Oteng-Ntim, E, Ayensah, B, Knight, M and Howard, J. 2015. Pregnancy outcome in patients with sickle cell disease in the UK – a national cohort comparing sickle cell anaemia HbSS with HbSC. *British Journal of Haematology*, *169*(1): 129–37.
55. Royal College of Obstetricians and Gynaecologists (ROOG). 2011. Green-top guideline no. 61: management of sickle cell disease in pregnancy [online]. Available at www.rcog. org.uk/globalassets/documents/guidelines/gtg_61.pdf. Accessed 4 August 2015.
56. Howard, J and Oteng-Ntim, E. 2012. The obstetric management of sickle cell disease. *Best Practice and Research Clinical Obstetrics and Gynaecology*, *26*(1): 25–36.
57. National Institute for health and Clinical Excellence (NICE). 2012. Sickle cell acute painful episode: management of an acute painful sickle cell episode in hospital. NICE clinical guideline 143. Available at www.nice.org.uk/guidance/cg143/evidence/full-guideline-pdf-18663 4333. Accessed 12 September 2017.
58. Howard, J, Hart, N, Roberts-Harewood, M, Cummins, M, Awogbade, M and Davis, B on behalf of the BCSH Committee. 2015. Guideline on the management of acute chest syndrome in sickle cell disease. *British Journal of Haematology*, *169*(4): 492–505.

Chapter 8

Assessment of the cardiac system

Introduction

Since 2000–2, cardiac conditions have been the leading cause of death in the UK among pregnant women and those who have recently given birth.[1] Advances in medical/surgical treatment has allowed more women with pre-existing cardiac conditions to embark on pregnancy. Lifestyle issues, in particular obesity, have contributed to an increase in acquired cardiac disease. In the most recent MBRRACE-UK report, the majority of women who died from cardiac disease had been undiagnosed with cardiac disease.[1] This presents a particular challenge for midwives, as the initial symptoms may arise due to the physiological changes in pregnancy, and therefore midwives may be the first health professionals to recognise these new symptoms.

In general, there are two types of cardiac disease: congenital (abnormalities in the heart; these may have been repaired or not) and acquired (largely ischaemic and related to lifestyle/family history). Maternal deaths from acquired disease are much higher in the UK. Both may be undiagnosed, but, if known about, a referral to a cardiologist is necessary.

Physiology

Physiological pregnancy adaptations are usually well-tolerated; however, if there is underlying cardiac disease, the increase in cardiac output may have a profound effect. An increase in both heart rate and blood volume contributes to a significant rise in cardiac output in pregnancy. The systolic blood pressure will remain about the same due to vasodilation of the peripheral blood vessels. The haemodynamic changes are mediated by increased levels of oestrogen, progesterone and prostaglandins, with endothelial derived relaxing factor (EDRF, nitric oxide) responsible for the earliest vasodilatory effects.[2] Box 8.1 gives a summary of the key cardiovascular changes in pregnancy. Further changes occur in labour and the postnatal period (see section entitled 'Changes to the cardiovascular system in labour and the postnatal period' in this chapter).

Clinical features of cardiac disorders

Predisposing/risk factors

Predisposing and/or risk factors are usually identified at booking by the midwife, and the knowledge of these can underpin suspicion of heart involvement if the woman presents with symptoms. Risks for cardiac disorders include:

- smoking history;
- obesity;
- family history of cardiac disease;
- other pre-existing medical conditions;
- increased age.

Signs and symptoms

Shortness of breath

Shortness of breath (SOB), also known as breathlessness, is one of the most common presenting symptoms for those with cardiac disease. However, it is also a common presenting symptom for many other conditions, including respiratory disease and sepsis, as well as being a normal pregnancy symptom (see Chapter 7 for discussion of how differentiation between pathological and physiological SOB may be made). Unexplained SOB should always be investigated, especially if increasing, or involving orthopnoea, paroxysmal nocturnal dyspnoea or syncope.

Level of consciousness and behaviour changes

Level of consciousness and mood state can be sensitive indicators of cardiac function.[6] Alternation of cardiac output will influence cerebral perfusion, and a reduction in cerebral perfusion can lead to drowsiness, confusion, agitation and reduced level of consciousness – and finally to unconsciousness.[7]

Alternatively, the woman may feel a sense of suffocation, become very frightened and anxious but not be hypoxic.[8]

Cyanosis

Cyanosis is usually considered a late sign of cardio-respiratory dysfunction; however, this is subject to considerable variability of assessment. It may be difficult to appreciate, in artificial lighting and in those of dark pigmented skin, when skin becomes dusky.

Chest pain

Chest pain (and pain in other sites) is a common presenting symptom for those with cardiac disease – see questions concerning assessment of this pain in Box 8.2.

Other common signs and symptoms

- Palpitations
- Murmur
- Syncope/collapse
- Peripheral oedema
- Irregular pulse
- Tachycardia
- Isolated systolic hypertension
- Polycythaemia
- Cough.

For many signs and symptoms, there may be other diagnoses, or indeed they may be only symptomatic of being pregnant. The midwife needs to evaluate signs and symptoms carefully to ensure referrals are made when necessary.

Changes to the cardiovascular system in labour and the postnatal period

Substantial increases in cardiac output in labour and the postnatal period make this a vulnerable time for those women with cardiac disease. Enhanced observation is vital at this time.

There is a 15% increase of the cardiac output in the first stage of labour and a 50% increase in the second stage.[3] This reaches a peak during contractions, when about 400 mls of additional blood is pushed into the circulation. Sympathetic nervous system response to pain and anxiety further elevates heart rate and blood pressure at this time.[5]

However, the biggest rise occurs immediately after the birth, when cardiac output increases by 60–80%. This rise is due to a number of factors: relief in pressure from the gravid uterus with subsequent improvement in venous return, transfusion of blood from placental bed back into the maternal circulation and loss of the extra vascular bed due to absence of placental blood flow. Excess blood loss and the use of drugs such as ergometrine that increase BP further complicate haemodynamic shifts affecting the heart at this time. Therefore, careful observation needs to be made of women who may be compromised by fluid swings, which could lead to congestive heart failure. O_2 saturation levels should be continuously monitored, as a reduction may indicate pulmonary oedema. Hypoxia increases pulmonary vascular resistance,[9] so oxygen administration may be required. It has been observed that, 1–2 hours postnatal, the cardiac output and stroke volume is still elevated, and there is evidence that changes in the haemodynamic status persist for some time into the puerperium.[10] CVP or arterial lines may be continued from labour or inserted to guide fluid administration and/or monitor the woman's condition immediately after birth.

Diuresis to get rid of extracellular fluid occurs between days two and five. Without this diuresis, pulmonary oedema can develop in women with pre-eclampsia or heart disease. Assessment of fluid balance will monitor these changes. Cardiac output gradually decreases to non-pregnant values by 6–12 weeks postnatally.[5]

Investigation, management and ongoing assessment of the cardiovascular system

ABC

- Airway: ensure a clear airway and position appropriately.
- Breathing: monitor respirations, attach pulse oximetry (reading can help determine clinical severity) and give oxygen as indicated.
- Circulation: cannulate appropriately, commence fluids according to the woman's needs and monitor pulse and BP.

History

The assessment of every woman contains a variety of questions that elicit a history, enabling a potential diagnosis and identifying areas where ongoing assessment is needed. Where cardiac conditions are suspected, the clinician will rely very strongly on analysis of pain symptoms in order to identify investigations that may be needed. They also provide areas where evaluation of progression, disappearance or even change of the pain can indicate whether treatments are effective or the condition is deteriorating. Some suggested questions to assess the chest pain are in Box 8.2.

Box 8.2 Questions to assess chest pain

- How did the pain begin (sudden onset/gradual/related to anything)?
- Does pain occur on effort/rest?
- Has it ever happened before?
- What is the character of the pain (dull, sharp, stabbing, diffuse, one small area, tearing, crushing)?
- Is area tender to palpation?
- Is pain continuous?
- Does anything make it better/worse?
- Has any drug/analgesia been taken?
- Does pain radiate anywhere (back, abdomen, arm)?
- Is pain affected by position (worse lying flat/relieved on leaning forward)?
- Are there associated symptoms (nausea/SOB/haemoptysis)?
- Are there risk factors?

Vital signs

It is very important to undertake vital sign monitoring regularly and chart on MEOWS (or specialty critical care charts), to ensure subtle changes are identified early. Regular and frequent assessment is necessary to identify deterioration in the woman's condition: increased pulse, worsening oedema, change in cardiac murmur, signs of cardiac failure such as crepitation at lung bases or raised jugular venous pressure or signs of infection should prompt rapid escalation of concerns. The regular and frequent recording of vital signs and observations of the ECG will also provide information that is especially important to evaluate the effect of new drugs if they are introduced.

Pulse

As well as identifying the rate, assessment should also be made for quality, regularity and equality.[7] A thready pulse can indicate poor cardiac output.

Blood pressure

A narrow pulse pressure, i.e. the difference between systolic and diastolic pressure (normal is 35–45 mmHg), suggests arterial vasoconstriction, potentially from cardiogenic shock or hypovolaemia.

Respirations

Careful observation of respiratory rate and quality, along with oxygen saturation readings, would be valuable to identify any deterioration in the woman's condition.

Temperature

Bacterial endocarditis and myocarditis may occur when there is damage to the cardio-vascular system from any cause, and it has been suggested that these conditions should always be considered when a cause of pyrexia is not immediately obvious.[11]

Blood tests

- Cardiac enzymes, in particular troponin (to diagnose MI), may need serial mea-surements;
- FBC (Hb for anaemia/WBC for infection);
- U&Es (electrolyte imbalance can cause arrhythmias);
- Renal function tests (elevation could indicate poor cardiac output);
- Clotting times;
- Lipids (cardiovascular risk factor);
- Amylase (rule out acute pancreatitis);
- CRP (assess inflammatory process);
- Capillary glucose assessment;
- ABGs if necessary;
- All cases of documented sinus tachycardia, SVT or atrial fibrillation or flutter should have thyroid function measured.[3]

Fluid balance

When cannulating, the state of the veins should be assessed: under-filled or collapsed veins could indicate hypovolaemia.

As it is possible the heart may not be working efficiently, the dangers of overload are clear. Fluid administration will depend on individual conditions and the physical state of the woman, but the midwife must ensure accurate fluid balance records are maintained, and hourly urine measurements are particularly important at this time. Fluid balance is vital post-delivery, and most deaths from cardiac disease occur at this time.[12] High dependency care should continue for 24–72 hours after delivery, as significant fluid shift can lead to congestive cardiac failure and, if spontaneous diuresis does not occur, pulmonary oedema may result.[13]

Midwifery considerations

VTE

Treatment of most women with heart disease includes anti-coagulant therapy, and this may have been discontinued for delivery of the baby. When prescribed to recommence, the midwife should ensure this takes place (teaching the woman to give LMWH injections if this is a new procedure). Meanwhile, the midwife needs to ensure she encourages preventative measures.[14] Although early mobilisation would be ideal, it may not be possible initially, and therefore it is important to ensure:

- wearing of correctly-fitting anti-embolic stockings (AES);
- deep-breathing exercises to encourage venous return;

- effective post-partum pain relief to enable mobility;
- intermittent pneumatic compression devices used during operative procedures and while immobile;
- adequate hydration.

Infection

Infection rates in the puerperium are directly related to the length and the number of interventions during labour, and a woman with cardiac disease may have received many interventions. Besides making sure strict asepsis is followed wherever appropriate, the midwife could also ensure the woman understands the importance of sleep and nutrition to efficient healing and building a healthy immune system.[15]

Psychological and social

If the woman was newly diagnosed with cardiac disease during pregnancy, she will need to be made aware of how to access appropriate ongoing care, and the importance of pre-conception care if she plans another pregnancy.

Investigations

Cardiac monitor

A bedside cardiac monitor (oscilloscope) provides a continuous display of the woman's ECG. See Box 8.3 concerning the set-up. Any deviation from normal sinus rhythm (see Figure 8.1) must be referred to an expert practitioner for evaluation.

Box 8.3 To set up an ECG monitor

- Explain/consent.
- Prep skin: ensure skin is dry, not greasy (use an alcohol swab if necessary).
- Attach electrodes:
  - red (right shoulder);
  - yellow (left shoulder);
  - green (left lower thorax);
  - (if five-lead: black right lower thorax, white chest).
- Switch on and ensure ECG is displaying clearly (the size of complex can be altered: if too low or too high, trace may be unclear and misinterpreted).
- Set alarms (according to local guidelines and the woman's condition).
- Ensure the screen is visible to healthcare staff.
- Document.

CHARACTERISTICS OF SINUS RHYTHM

Basic evaluation includes appearance and time between each component.

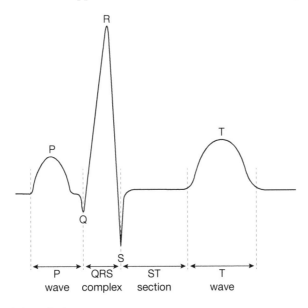

Figure 8.1 Normal sinus rhythm

Source: Philip Woodrow. 2016. *Nursing acutely ill adults*. Oxford, UK: Routledge.

- P wave: atrial contraction (depolarisation of atria);
- QRS complex: pressure in ventricle rises prior to ejection (depolarisation of ventricles);
- T wave: ventricle pressure falls (repolarisation of ventricles).

Ectopics are isolated beats from abnormal pacemakers, and may appear randomly or regularly in a normal sinus rhythm trace (see Figure 8.2). Referral for expert opinion is always necessary, but, if only occasional, they may be benign. A common cause is electrolyte imbalance, in particular potassium imbalance, but calcium and magnesium imbalances can also cause ectopics,[16] and these should be treated. Frequent premature ectopics are also usually treated as they can progress to dysrhythmias.[16]

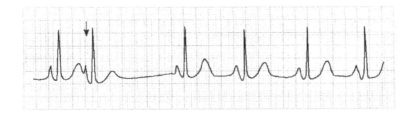

Figure 8.2 Ectopics

Source: Philip Woodrow. 2012. *Intensive care nursing*, 3rd edition. Oxford, UK: Routledge.

Electrocardiogram (ECG)

A 12-lead ECG is a time/voltage graph of myocardial electrical activity,[16] recording changes in electrical activity during each part of the cardiac cycle, observed from 12 different views.[17] The interpretation of the electrical activity of the heart is expressed through the use of ten electrodes, which are attached to the limbs and chest, and which can record in real time.[18] The 12-lead ECG is recognised as the current medical standard for the identification, analysis and confirmation of many cardiac abnormalities,[19] and is a standard test carried out in maternity care whenever a woman presents with symptoms that could be related to cardiac conditions. However, as with all individual tests, clinical history and physical examination are also vital.

Ten electrodes are placed on the skin: one on each ankle and wrist, and six across the chest (see Figure 8.3). Electrodes are connected to wires (identified for placement), which feed into the ECG device.

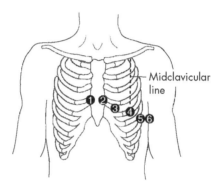

Figure 8.3 Placement of chest leads for ECG

Source: Philip Woodrow. 2012. *Intensive care nursing*, 3rd edition. Oxford, UK: Routledge.

Echocardiogram (transthoracic/transoesophageal)

Many cardiac disorders can be identified by clinical examination and history, but most need an echocardiogram to confirm.[20] An echocardiogram is a diagnostic imaging procedure, which uses high-frequency ultrasound waves to view the heart.[18] Echo-cardiograms can be transthoracic or transoesophageal. Transthoracic is considered technically more difficult in pregnancy with the pressure from the fetus, breast engorgement and rotation of the heart;[21] however, it is non-invasive so is far more acceptable to women.

Transoesophageal echocardiography is an ultrasound technique that involves introducing a probe on the end of a flexible gastroscope-like probe, which can be manoeuvred within the oesophagus and stomach, close to the heart.

Echocardiograms can measure cardiac function and structure, identifying regional wall abnormalities that occur in myocardial ischaemia and necrosis.[22] They can also be useful to diagnose aortic dissection and pulmonary emboli.[22] Serial echocardiograms can be used for assessment and/or surveillance of known pathologies.[18]

Chest X-ray

An X-ray may be useful to potentially identify pulmonary oedema, spontaneous pneumothorax and/or increased cardiac ratio as a result of left ventricular dilation, but mainly it is used to exclude other potential causes of chest pain.[23] Shielding of the uterus would be routinely carried out, but it is suggested that a chest X-ray should not be withheld if it is an investigation that is needed, as it only exposes the fetus to a very small fraction of the maximum recommended exposure in pregnancy.[3]

Additional investigations

24-hour Holter ECG

Rarely carried out in pregnancy, but a common postnatal test, a 24-hour heart rate and rhythm (Holter ECG) record is made when there is a suspicion of significant arrhythmias, or complaints of syncope or prolonged palpitations.[21]

Cardiac MRI (magnetic resonance imaging)

A cardiac MRI is mainly used for diagnosis of diseases of the aorta and complex congenital heart disease.[24] Although safety during pregnancy has not yet been totally established, no harmful effects on the fetus have been raised.[24] However, imaging should be avoided during the first trimester if possible.[25]

Cardiac CT (computed tomography)

A computed tomography (CT) is a diagnostic imaging tool that uses X-ray beams in multiple directions, creating image slices that can be used to reconstruct two-dimensional (2D) and three-dimensional (3D) images. It can be used to confirm aortic dissection if MRI and transoesophageal echocardiography are not available.[24] Safety issues vary with gestation, and current recommendations are for use only when benefits clearly outweigh potential risks.[24]

Coronary angiogram

Angiography (catheter introduced via the femoral or brachial artery) can be used to assess the coronary arteries, or treat them using an inflatable balloon to widen them – a stent can then be put in place if necessary. There is a radiation risk to the fetus, but this can be reduced by various methods such as lead shielding of the mother's abdomen and back and reducing screening time.[26]

Specific cardiac conditions

Arrhythmias

Although some arrhythmias are benign, others have the potential for harm: some are immediately life-threatening, and some may adversely influence cardiac function. Acute arrhythmias are often triggered by infection, myocardial hypoxia or abnormal blood chemistry (especially potassium, magnesium and calcium). They may be a preliminary sign of further deterioration (either because of the arrhythmia or because of the underlying cardiac disease causing the arrhythmia). Other signs and symptoms such as hypotension (systolic < 90), pallor, sweating, cold/clammy extremities, confusion and impaired consciousness, should be evaluated.

Interpretation of the range of arrhythmias is beyond the usual role of the midwife. However, midwives should be able to recognise abnormalities and ensure each and any arrhythmia is brought to the attention of a skilled and experienced member of the MDT for assessment and treatment if necessary.

Aortic dissection

Pregnancy gives rise to changes in structure of the vessel walls. This includes an increase in aortic size and compliance. Oestrogens can interfere with collagen deposition, weakening vessel walls and predisposing to dissection such as aortic dissection.[27] This can be a particular problem for women with Marfan syndrome, which is a disorder of connective tissue.

Women with genetic abnormalities, especially Marfan, Ehlers-Danlos syndrome and Loeys-Dietz syndrome, are known to be at risk of aortic dissection, and, if diagnosed before pregnancy, need referral to cardiologists and will be closely monitored. However, many women with these conditions have not been previously diagnosed, and there are also women who have a dissection from the effect of pregnancy.[28]

Therefore, an aortic root dissection can present in otherwise healthy women, and signs and symptoms such as central chest or interscapular pain, a wide pulse pressure (mainly secondary to systolic hypertension) and a new cardiac murmur must prompt referral to a cardiologist and appropriate imaging.[29] Although rupture can happen at any time in pregnancy, the time of greatest risk is labour and the immediate postnatal period, when cardiac output is increased. Hypertension increases the risk of dissection, and systolic BP needs to be carefully monitored and controlled.

The clinical presentation of aortic dissection includes shock, dyspnoea, cyanosis, anxiety and a feeling of impending doom. In the early stages, there may only be an elevated BP.[30] A ripping/tearing sensation has been described, and if the dissection extends into the arterial tree, neurovascular symptoms (headache, visual disturbances) as well as pulseless limbs and severe, sudden onset, localised chest and back pain may occur.[1]

There is much overlap of symptoms between respiratory disorders (primarily PE) and cardiac dissection, and the MBRRACE confidential enquiries[1] described cases where, following the exclusion of a diagnosis of PE, women were discharged home, without an explanation for the symptoms, where they then died.

Acute coronary syndrome

Acute coronary syndrome is the umbrella term that covers different presentations of acute myocardial ischaemia, from unstable angina to myocardial infarction, including acute coronary artery dissection. Myocardial ischaemia is reduced circulation of oxygenated blood to the heart muscle caused by atherosclerosis. Atherosclerosis is a progressive, degenerating arterial disease that leads to gradual blockage of affected vessels. Blockages caused by atheromatous plaques, a feature of the disease, can be complicated by clot formation. The tissue beyond these narrow points becomes ischaemic, and pain caused by these blockages is called angina. When a coronary artery becomes blocked it is known as myocardial infarction.

The numbers of women with acute coronary syndromes in pregnancy are increasing, with a high risk of mortality and significant morbidity.[26]

Myocardial infarction (MI)

Although about 50% of women report traditional symptoms for an MI (crushing chest pain, radiating to jaw and left arm), many female symptoms differ from the classic ones normal for men. For example, women may have unspecific chest pain, or pain outside the chest region (upper limbs, neck, jaw and stomach), dizziness, SOB and/or anxiety.[23] Other complications to reaching the correct diagnosis include:

- Age: young women are treated with less suspicion, especially if breathless rather than complaining of acute chest pain.[23]
- Normal or non-specific ECG findings: these may not be classic features for MI or may be transient ischaemia.
- The inhibiting effects of pain and fear: especially when pregnant and therefore possibly focussing on the wellbeing of the fetus.

Midwives must ensure there is a low threshold to investigate women with chest pain.[26]

MI diagnosis:[18]

- History of ischaemia;
- Serial ECG changes;
- Raised serum cardiac enzymes (especially troponin).

Coronary artery dissection (CAD)

In pregnancy, coronary artery dissection (or spontaneous coronary artery dissection: SCAD) occurs commonly in late pregnancy or the early puerperal period. The highest incidence is found to occur immediately after delivery and this is suggested to be caused by a combination of elevated cardiac output, increased total blood volume and sheering forces during labour with increasing catecholamine stimulus due to pain.[12] There is also a close association with connective tissue disorders.

Valvular heart disease/valve replacement

Those women with untreated cardiac valve disease may become symptomatic for the first time in pregnancy, due to increasing fluid circulation. However, those women who have previously received a prosthetic valve may also have complications in pregnancy, and should have a cardiac referral as soon as possible. A recent study[1] into morbidity following pregnancy/delivery identified serious maternal complications, including valve thrombosis, CVA and endocarditis.

Midwives caring for women with prosthetic cardiac valves must ensure there is specialist cardiology input, especially in the areas of anticoagulation and potential antibiotic use.

SADS/MNH (sudden arrhythmic cardiac death with a morphologically normal heart)

SADS is the diagnosis when a sudden unexpected cardiac death occurs and all other causes are excluded following an autopsy. This follows a cardiac arrest, and it is thought that some may survive with prompt resuscitation. The cause is presumed to be due to arrhythmia.

SADS was the commonest cause of cardiac death in the most recent confidential enquiries.[1] In this analysis of the women who died, no clear predisposing/risk factors were identified, and it appears there were no obvious warning signs.

A genetic component has been identified in some cases, and therefore the family of those who die need referrals. It is also possible that a woman may book with the history of a sudden unexplained cardiac death in her family, and these women should be referred for investigation.

Peripartum cardiomyopathy (PPCM)

Peripartum cardiomyopathy is a condition that is specific to pregnancy and often has a very insidious onset. This can be defined as an idiopathic cardiomyopathy presenting with heart failure secondary to left ventricle systolic dysfunction towards the end of pregnancy or in the months following delivery, where no other cause of heart failure is found. It is a diagnosis of exclusion.[31] The incidence may be increasing.[4]

Peripartum cardiomyopathy may be mild/self-limiting or can lead to severe heart failure, which can result in residual disease[32] and/or death.[33] In one study, the time from first symptoms to diagnosis varied between 3 and 190 days.[20]

Predisposing/risk factors may include age over 30,[34] obesity, multifetal pregnancies and/or hypertensive complications, but there may also be no identifiable risk factors.[12]

The main symptoms of PPCM include fatigue, SOB, fluid retention, chest tightness, tremor, dizziness, syncope, restlessness, tingly body, reduced urine output, orthopnoea, breathlessness with activity and emotional symptoms such as acute anxiety. Symptoms may intensify as time goes on, but, as soon as the midwife suspects these changes, urgent referral is required. An early diagnosis can prevent complications and improve outcomes.[35] The referral will generate the following tests:

- Chest X-ray (cardiomegaly, pulmonary oedema, pleural effusion);
- 12-lead ECG;
- Echocardiography.

PPCM is a diagnosis of exclusion, so a full range of cardiac blood assessments are necessary,[33] including cardiac enzymes, thyroid function tests and CRP.

Ongoing assessment will include continuous ECG, very frequent recording of vital signs, continuous oxygen saturation monitoring, early and perhaps multiple IV access and strict fluid balance. If antenatal, CTG abnormalities may be the first sign of maternal poor oxygenation and circulatory compromise. The mode and timing of delivery will be dependent on the degree of compromise in the mother and condition of the fetus.

It is estimated that about half of women will have a full recovery.[4] However, even if recovery appears complete, there is a high risk of recurrence in subsequent pregnancies,[36] and women need to be aware to obtain reliable contraception and seek appropriate assessment and counselling before considering another pregnancy. Follow-up cardiac care is usual.

References

1. Vause, S, Clarke, B, Thorne, S, James, R, Lucas, S, Youd, E, Kinsella, M and Knight, M on behalf of the MBRRACE-UK cardiovascular chapter writing group. 2016. Lessons on cardiovascular disease. In: Knight, M, Nour, M, Tuffnell, D, Kenyon, S, Shakespeare, J, Brocklehurst, P and Kurinczuk, JJ (eds) on behalf of MBRRACE-UK. *Saving lives, improving mothers' care: surveillance of maternal deaths in the UK 2012–2014 and lessons learned to inform maternity care from the UK and Ireland Confidential Enquiries into Maternal Deaths and Morbidity 2009–2014*. Oxford, UK: National Perinatal Epidemiology Unit, University of Oxford, pp. 33–68.
2. Bothamley, J and Boyle, M. 2009. *Medical conditions affecting pregnancy and childbirth*. Oxford, UK: Radcliffe.
3. Nelson-Piercy, C. 2015. *Handbook of obstetric medicine*. Boca Raton, FL: CRC Press.
4. Lewey, J and Haythe, J. 2014. Cardiomyopathy in pregnancy. *Seminars in Perinatology*, 38(5): 309–17.
5. Blackburn, ST. 2013. *Maternal, fetal and neonatal physiology*. Maryland Heights, MO: Saunders.
6. Reynolds, A. 1999. *Critical and high acuity nursing care*. New York: Thompson Learning.
7. Smith, G. 2003. *ALERT: acute life-threatening events, recognition and treatment*. Portsmouth, UK: University of Portsmouth.
8. Moore, T and Woodrow, P. 2009. *High dependency nursing care: observation, intervention and support for level 2 patients*. London: Routledge.
9. Rosenthal, E and Nelson-Piercy, C. 2000. Value of inhaled nitric oxide in Eisenmenger syndrome during pregnancy. *American Journal of Obstetrics and Gynecology*, 183(3): 781–2.
10. Ramsay, M. 2006. Management of the puerperium in women with heart disease. In: Steer, P, Gatzoulis, M and Baker, P (eds). *Heart disease and pregnancy*. London: RCOG, pp. 299–312.
11. Billington, M and Stevenson, M. 2007. *Critical care in childbearing for midwives*. Oxford, UK: Blackwell Publishing.
12. Paterson-Brown, S and Howell, C. 2014. *Managing obstetric emergencies and trauma: the MOET course manual*. Cambridge, UK: Cambridge University Press.
13. Tomlinson, M. 2011. Cardiac disease. In: James, D, Steer, P, Weiner, C and Gonik, B (eds). *High risk pregnancy: management options*. St Louis, MO: Elsevier Saunders, pp. 627–55.
14. Bothamley, J. 2017. Thromboembolism in pregnancy. In: Boyle, M (ed.). *Emergencies around childbirth*. Boca Raton, FL: CRC Press, pp. 55–76.
15. Bothamley, J and Boyle, M. 2015. *Infections affecting pregnancy and childbirth*. London: Radcliffe.
16. Woodrow, P. 2012. *Intensive care nursing*. London: Routledge
17. Dutton, H and Finch, J (eds). 2018. *Acute and critical care nursing at a glance*. London: John Wiley & Sons.

18. Camm, CF and Camm, AJ (eds). 2016. *Clinical guide to cardiology*. Oxford, UK: Wiley-Blackwell.
19. Jevon, P and Ewens, B. 2012. *Monitoring the critically ill patient*. Oxford, UK: Blackwell Publishing.
20. Patel, H, Berg, M, Barasa, A, Begley, C and Schaufelberger, M. 2016. Symptoms in women with peripartum cardiomyopathy: a mixed method study. *Midwifery, 32*: 14–20.
21. Elliott, C, Sliwa, K and Burton, R. 2014. Pregnancy and cardiac disease. *South African Medical Journal, 104*(9): 641–6.
22. Van de Werf, F, Ardissino, D, Betriu, A, Cokkinos, DV, Falk, E, Fox, KA . . . and Wijns, W on behalf of Task Force on the Management of Acute Myocardial Infarction of the European Society of Cardiology. 2003. Management of acute myocardial infarction in patients presenting with ST-segment elevation. *European Heart Journal, 24*(1): 28–66.
23. Albarran, J and Tagney, J. 2007. *Chest pain: advanced assessment and management skills*. Oxford, UK: Blackwell Publishing
24. Waksmonski, C. 2014. Cardiac imaging and functional assessment in pregnancy. *Seminars in Perinatology, 38*(5): 240–4.
25. Regitz-Zagrosek, V, Lundqvist, CB, Borghi, C, Cifkova, R, Ferreira, R, Foidart, J-M . . . and Torracca, L on behalf of the European Society of Gynecology (ESG), the Association for European Paediatric Cardiology (AEPC) and the German Society for Gender Medicine (DGesGM). 2011. Guidelines on the management of cardiovascular diseases during pregnancy: the task force on the management of cardiovascular diseases during pregnancy of the European Society of Cardiology (ECS). *European Heart Journal, 32*: 3147–97
26. Fryearson, J and Adamson, D. 2014. Heart disease in pregnancy: ischaemic heart disease. *Best Practice and Research Clinical Obstetrics and Gynaecology, 28*(4): 551–62.
27. Bonow, RO, Carabello, BA, Chatterjee, K, de Leon, AC Jr, Faxon, DP, Freed, MD . . . and Shanewise, JS. 2006. Guidelines for the management of patients with valvular heart disease: executive summary: a report of the American College of Cardiology/American Heart Association Task Force on Practice. *Circulation, 114*: 1–78.
28. Yuan, S. 2013. Aortic dissection during pregnancy: a difficult clinical scenario. *Clinical Cardiology, 36*(10): 576–84.
29. Royal College of Obstetricians and Gynaecologists (RCOG). 2011. Green-top guideline no. 56: maternal collapse in pregnancy and the puerperium. London: RCOG.
30. Yee, C. 2004. Aortic dissection: the tear that kills. *Journal of Nursing Management, 35*(2): 25–32.
31. Sliwa, K, Hilfiker-Kleiner, D, Petrie, MC, Mebazaa, A, Pieske, B, Buchmann, E . . . and McMurray, JJ. 2010. Current state of knowledge on aetiology, diagnosis, management and therapy of peripartum cardiomyopathy: a position statement from the Heart Failure Association of the European Society of Cardiology Working Group on peripartum cardiomyopathy. *European Journal of Heart Failure, 12*(8) 767–78.
32. Shani, H, Kuperstein, R and Berlin, A. 2015. Peripartum cardiomyopathy: risk factors, characteristics and long-term follow-up. *Journal of Perinatal Medicine, 43*(1): 95–101.
33. Stamatelatou, M, Walker, F and Pandya, B. 2015. A contemporary review of peripartum cardiomyopathy. *British Journal of Midwifery, 23*(6): 394–400.
34. Deas, J. 2017. Peripartum cardiomyopathy. *MIDIRS Midwifery Digest, 27*(2): 197–200.
35. Elkayam, U, Goland, S, Pieper, PG and Silverside, CK. 2016. High-risk cardiac disease in pregnancy: part II. *Journal of the American College of Cardiology, 68*(5): 502–16.
36. Fett, J, Shad, T and McNamara, D. 2015. Why do some recovered peripartum cardiomyopathy mothers experience heart failure with a subsequent pregnancy? *Current Treatment Options in Cardiovascular Medicine, 17*(1): 354.

Chapter 9

Assessment of the neurological system

Introduction

In the UK, 11% of maternal mortality is related to diseases affecting the central nervous system.[1,2,3] Neurological disorders causing death included subarachnoid haemorrhage, intracerebral haemorrhage, cerebral thrombosis and epilepsy. Fortunately, life-threatening neurological emergencies are still relatively rare, although may be related to previous underlying disease or be linked to the physiological changes in pregnancy. Pre-eclampsia is known to have a neurological manifestation in some women, the most obvious being an eclamptic seizure.

Competence in basic neurological assessment is an important midwifery skill that enables early detection and management of neurological and medical emergencies. In particular, assessment of behaviour change and level of consciousness, assessment of headache and management of seizures are important. The response to a neurological emergency will require a multidisciplinary approach, involving close liaison between the neurology, neurosurgery and obstetric teams. Anaesthetic, critical outreach, ITU and radiology staff are some further key members required to give such specialist care. As always, the midwife may be involved in initial assessment and instigate urgent referral, and should remain involved for essential ongoing family support.

Physiology

Cerebral perfusion is the term used to indicate the supply of oxygenated blood to the brain. The blood supply to the brain is both essential and complex. An adequate mean arterial pressure (blood pressure) needs to ensure adequate cerebral perfusion. Cerebral auto-regulation usually controls intracranial pressure.

Space inside the skull (intracranial) is limited. In other parts of the body, when there is bleeding or an increase of the fluid within the body compartments, there is pressure on tissue and the area distends. The brain is enclosed in a rigid box (the skull), and, as such, the volume that can be contained within it is fixed. If there is any bleeding or increase in fluid (oedema), this will raise intracranial pressure and start compressing brain tissue, causing damage to brain cells.[4] Factors that affect intracranial pressure (ICP) will affect cerebral perfusion and have the potential to contribute to neurological damage. Signs of raised ICP are headache, neck stiffness, slow pulse and high blood pressure.

The main components inside the skull and the factors that may affect ICP are:

- Brain substance: tumours and blood clots can add to brain tissue increasing pressure.
- Cerebrospinal fluid (CSF): CSF protects the brain and spinal cord from injury. Approximately 80–150 ml of CSF circulates continuously in the subarachnoid space around the brain and in the spinal cord. It is produced by a network of capillaries known as the choroid plexus in the walls of the ventricles, and is absorbed back into the blood by finger-like projections in the arachnoid mater. CSF fluid can increase pressure if there is a blockage to the usual drainage.[5] This can happen with meningitis. Dural tap during epidural pain relief causes a reduction in CSF, leading to headache.
- Cerebral blood vessels and the blood contained within these vessels: a rise in arterial carbon dioxide can lead to increased cerebral vasodilation. If the pressure within blood vessels rises too high or too rapidly, this can lead to a haemorrhagic stroke. Raised systolic blood pressure > 160 mmHg, associated with PET, has been identified as a cause of maternal death.[6]
- Extracellular fluid: the fluid within brain tissue is affected by electrolyte imbalance. These imbalances, particularly changes in sodium levels, can affect cerebral function, and levels need to be corrected slowly. Extracellular fluid can increase in response to brain injury and careful fluid management will be part of care to prevent further complications.

Neurological assessment by the midwife

Once identified, women with significant neurological impairment will be cared for in a specialist unit, although midwives and obstetricians will still form part of the multidisciplinary team. However, all midwives need to be able to assess significant acute neurological changes to enable early intervention. This will be a rare event in maternity care, so all that is required is a basic assessment that identifies any deteriorating condition and ensures specialist help is accessed urgently. Despite the rarity, conditions specific to pregnancy predispose women to developing neurological problems, and these conditions can be identified early, making prevention of neurological disorders a priority. Changes in a woman's behaviour may be the first indication of neurological impairment and all staff should be encouraged to report any worrying changes observed by themselves or the woman's family. AVPU assessment should be performed and recorded at every regular MEOWS chart assessment.

Prompt recognition of signs and symptoms of PET and control of high systolic blood pressures are essential to preventing morbidity and mortality from stroke. Effective risk assessment and thromboprophylaxis for women at risk of thromboembolism will help reduce deaths associated with cerebral vein thrombosis. The assessment for these conditions is part of the everyday role of the midwife.

Midwives will commonly assess neurological function through:

- changes in mood or behaviour;
- AVPU assessment of level of consciousness;
- review of headache and visual disturbances;
- limb movement, motor response, loss of sensation;
- regular observations of respiratory rate, oxygen saturations, pulse, blood pressure and temperature;
- midwifery head-to-toe examination to elicit general wellbeing of mother and fetus/newborn.

More advanced neurological assessment by midwives with specialist skills in critical care may include:

- Glasgow Coma Scale assessment;
- pupil size, shape, equality and reaction to light.

Behaviour

A change in behaviour, such as agitation, restlessness, drowsiness and confusion, is often the first sign of possible neurological impairment. The midwife may notice this but should also be careful to note comments made by the woman's family as well. Changes in behaviour may include:[7]

- aggressiveness or confusion – linked to acidosis, but could also be evident with abnormalities of the blood sugar (e.g. hypoglycaemia in a diabetic);
- altered cognition;
- motor impairment (dribbling), difficulty swallowing (dysphagia), difficulty with communication (dysphasia), weakness;
- hallucinations.

Regular observations and midwifery head-to-toe assessment

Regular observations of pulse, blood pressure, respiratory rate and oxygen saturations should be carried out and documented on a MEOWS chart. This feeds into the ABC assessment. A usual head-to-toe midwifery assessment should also be included once the requirements of ABC are attended to. This assessment could pick up other key features that will provide information about underlying conditions. Is the woman's skin cold and clammy (shock)? Are there any unusual rashes (meningitis)? Oedema (PET)? Diarrhoea (sepsis)? Urine testing will also give valuable information regarding ill health, such as the presence of protein, glucose or ketones.

Observation of limb tone and movement would be included in the information gathered on a head-to-toe examination.

A loss of consciousness may be accompanied by changes in vital signs. Raised intracranial pressure from internal bleeding or brain swelling can put pressure on the cardiovascular and respiratory centres located in the brain stem. This may cause the heart rate to slow and blood pressure to rise. Respiratory effort may diminish. Box 9.1 lists further investigations that will aid assessment and diagnosis.

Box 9.1 Investigations for neurological symptoms

- Laboratory blood tests: FBC, uric acid, LFTs, random blood sugar, CRP;
- Computerised tomography (CT) scan;
- Magnetic resonance imaging (MRI);
- Lumbar puncture.

AVPU assessment

Basic neurological AVPU assessment is included in the Modified Early Obstetric Warning Score (MEOWS) (see Table 9.1). AVPU is a useful quick, general initial assessment, but should be followed up with Glasgow Coma Scale (GCS) assessment in all cases where the woman is deemed not to be 'alert'.

Table 9.1 AVPU assessment

Alert	MEOWS 0
V – responds to **verbal** stimuli	MEOWS 1
P – responds to **painful** stimuli	MEOWS 2
Unresponsive	MEOWS 3

Midwives will usually recognise a woman who is alert and acting normally.

If any woman is not alert, her response to verbal stimuli should be assessed by simply talking to her, saying 'Hello' or perhaps asking 'How are you?'. The woman may respond to voice (such as turning her head), but if her response is not coherent, that is cause for concern and may indicate neurological problems. Any AVPU score below 'Alert' should prompt further assessment, such as checking the GCS, checking the blood sugar level and seeking a medical opinion. The midwife should carry out a general midwifery assessment and perform a set of observations.

Assessment of the woman's response to pain should only be carried out if the woman is unresponsive to voice, although the midwife should already have identified the need for urgent medical assistance at this point. Reduced or altered consciousness level is not an early warning sign: it is a red flag symptom that indicates established illness.[6] Initial AVPU assessment of her response to pain would involve vigorously shaking the woman's shoulders.[7] GCS assessment of pain uses more specific locations to elicit the specific level of deficit. Being unresponsive is generally a very poor sign, indicating loss of consciousness and significant, serious pathology.

A limitation of AVPU in terms of triggering an alert is that it doesn't include a score for behavioural changes such as agitation or development of significant headache. Confusion and aggression might arise if the diabetic woman has a low blood sugar or as a feature of shock, so assessment of other factors such as a blood sugar level, pulse, BP respiratory rate and saturations need to be made as well. As always, scoring systems need to be used alongside effective general clinical assessment.

The frequency of AVPU assessment will be determined by clinical factors. Where there are no identified neurological concerns, AVPU assessment will be made at the same frequency as indicated for general MEOWS assessment – around every 4–8 hours. If there is new concern about neurological deficit, such as a reduced AVPU score, significant headache, confusion or agitation, the frequency will need to be increased to every 5–15 minutes with constant direct observation of the woman. The woman 'sleeping' should not be a reason not to perform the test when it is indicated, as sleepiness is in itself a sign of neurological impairment and dangerous deterioration of her condition could be missed.

Some specialist maternity critical care units may use a neurological observation chart, although where a woman is requiring such assessment she is likely to be moved into an acute critical care unit. A neurological observation chart would include a record of the GCS, BP and heart rate, pupil size and reaction and limb movement. The midwife can keep a record of these observations regardless of a chart or not, while awaiting transfer.

Limb movement

Focal neurologic signs or deficits are impairments of nerve function in the brain or spinal cord that affect a specific region of the body. Weakness in a limb, partial loss of voluntary movement and loss of sensation are examples of symptoms.

Evidence of spontaneous limb movements, tone and reflexes should be observed. Are they equal on both sides? If movement seems diminished, assess response to painful stimulus. One-sided limb weakness suggests intracranial injury. Remember that women will normally have reduced bilateral motor leg function in relation to multiple epidural top-ups and spinal anaesthesia.

Glasgow Coma Scale

GCS indicates level of consciousness by determining the degree of (increasing) stimulation that is required to elicit a response using three different assessments:

- eye opening
- best verbal response
- best motor response.

See Table 9.2 for elements and scoring of the Glasgow Coma Scale. The maximum score is 15, with 4 for eyes opening spontaneously, 5 when verbal response shows

Table 9.2 Elements and scoring of the Glasgow Coma Scale[8]

Eye opening		Best verbal response		Best motor response	
Spontaneously	4	Orientated	5	Obeys commands	6
To speech	3	Confused	4	Localising	5
To pressure	2	Words	3	Normal flexion (withdrawal)	4
None	1	Sounds	2	Abnormal flexion	3
		None	1	Extension	2
				None	1

that the woman is orientated and 6 when she is able to obey commands regarding motor response. No response in each category scores 1, so the minimum score is 3.[4]

Further detailed instruction on how to perform the GCS can be found at www. glasgowcomascale.org/, which includes a useful video. Further reading is suggested at the end of this chapter.

Pupil reaction

Pupil size and response to light is a useful assessment of neurological function that can be performed by the midwife, although this would be an uncommon assessment to be undertaken by midwives, even in a critical care setting. Pupil reactions are controlled by the third cranial nerve and the brainstem. Normally, the pupils dilate rapidly in darkness and then will constrict rapidly in response to a bright torchlight. Under ambient light the pupils should appear the same size.

Loss of consciousness

A state of unconsciousness can be sudden when there is inadequate oxygen or glucose getting to the brain tissue, or can manifest as a gradual decline. The likelihood of

---

Box 9.2 List of possible causes for unconsciousness that may occur in a maternity care setting[9]

- Hypoxia;
- Failure of circulation: hypovolaemic shock following PPH, APH or myocardial infarction;
- Anaphylaxis;
- Rupture or occlusion of cerebral vessels as in subarachnoid haemorrhage, cerebral vein thrombosis;
- Hypoglycaemia;

- Hyperglycaemia: ketoacidosis;
- Disorders of thyroid function;
- Raised intracranial pressure: e.g. caused by brain tumours;
- Drugs, alcohol or poisoning;
- Sepsis;
- Following seizure;
- Meningitis, encephalitis.

permanent disability increases with the period of unconsciousness. A state of unconsciousness is an emergency. See Box 9.2 for a list of possible causes for unconsciousness that may occur in a maternity care setting. Principles of ABCDE assessment and intervention are required: see Box 9.3.

Box 9.3 Checklist of midwifery assessment and intervention in cases of loss of consciousness

Many actions will be done simultaneously once staff respond to an emergency call for help. In cases of cardiac and/or respiratory arrest, follow the resuscitation guidelines for adult resuscitation.[10]

Call for help: emergency peri-arrest team and emergency obstetric team in hospital.

A: *Airway*: a woman with a reduced level of consciousness is more likely to obstruct her airway and is at risk of aspiration. Tilt the head posteriorly to straighten and slightly extend the neck, and gently lift the chin upward. Apply jaw thrust as required. An oropharyngeal airway may be helpful.

If it is established that she is not in cardiac/respiratory arrest, move the woman into the recovery position.

B: *Breathing*: administer oxygen via a rebreathing face mask if spontaneously breathing.

C: *Circulation*: check uterus is contracted and observe for any obvious bleeding.

A full set of observations required: temperature, heart rate, respiratory rate BP and oxygen saturations. Record on MEOWS chart and repeat at frequent intervals.

Gain IV access (two wide-bore cannulae).

IV fluids, as per medical instructions: be aware that, while fluid administration is often helpful, in some cases, such as PET, it can be detrimental.

D: *Disability*: assess and record AVPU frequently to assess any level of recovery.

E: *Exposure*: Head-to-toe assessment to help identify any causes for unconsciousness, stage of pregnancy and fetal wellbeing.

Send a range of laboratory tests. Check the blood sugar at the bedside (see discussion on ketoacidosis).

Other assessments/interventions:

- Monitoring the fetus;
- Catheterisation – measure hourly urine output, and dipstick catheter specimen of urine for protein and ketones;
- Medications as per medical instructions;
- Documentation;
- Psychological support of family.

Headache

The most common headache in pregnancy is a simple tension headache. Tension headaches are thought to be due to muscle contraction and are often related to periods of stress. Relaxation, rest, fluids and a simple analgesic will relieve symptoms. Migraine is a more serious headache that can be quite debilitating. Migraines usually improve in pregnancy, but often return postnatally when oestrogen concentrations fall.[11] Features of a migraine can include:[12]

- a throbbing, unilateral severe headache;
- visual prodromal symptoms: women see 'jagged lines';
- nausea and vomiting;
- photophobia or noise sensitivity.

A particularly debilitating migraine, known as hemiplegic migraine, can cause temporary muscle weakness on one side of the body, and partial or complete loss of vision. This loss of function can last several hours and differentiating this from features of a stroke is challenging. Very rarely, hemiplegic migraine does lead to stroke in pregnancy.[12]

Headaches are very common in pregnancy and only a small proportion will require detailed assessment and referral. An estimated 40% of women will have a headache in the postpartum period.[11] However, on every occasion that a woman complains of a headache, the midwife should take a careful history and perform an examination. The key issue for the midwife when a woman complains of a headache is to distinguish between a primary headache (tension or migraine) and a headache caused by secondary reasons, some of which indicate deteriorating neurological function (see Table 9.3). As the features of migraine overlap with more serious neurological impairment, the midwife is recommended to ask for further medical assessment in women who present

Table 9.3 Secondary causes of headache[12,9,11]

Possible causes of headaches	Features	Actions and investigations
Post-dural puncture headache (PDPH), related to epidural insertion	Onset usually within 24 hours of insertion of epidural. Worse when upright, may note relief within 10–15 minutes of lying down. Often associated with neck stiffness but may be associated with other neurological symptoms.	Refer to anaesthetist. Diagnosis by history and exclusion of other causes. Conservative management includes lying flat, analgesia, thromboprophylaxis, keeping hydrated and increasing caffeine intake. Consider epidural blood patch.
Drug-related headache	Some antihypertensive medications, particularly Nifedipine and Hydralazine, can give rise to headaches. May also occur with persistent use of analgesics.	Refer for medical review of medication.

continued

Table 9.3 continued

Possible causes of headaches	Features	Actions and investigations
Pre-eclampsia/ hypertension	Headaches may be severe and can be accompanied by visual disturbances, including flashing lights. Usually associated with other features of PET, such as hypertension, proteinuria, epigastric pain. May be linked to antihypertensive medication. Severe headache in context of fulminating PET may indicate intracerebral haemorrhage.	Urgent referral for step-up DAU review, including review by obstetrician. Assessment of BP, urinalysis, oedema, fetal wellbeing – including symphysis fundal height measurement – and other symptoms of PET should be recorded by the midwife. PET blood tests: FBC, U&Es, renal and liver function tests and measurement of urinary protein : creatinine ratio (PCR).
Subarachnoid haemorrhage	Sudden, severe and often felt in the occipital region – known as a 'thunderclap' headache. May have altered conscious level, confusion or coma.	Urgent referral. ABC assessment and response. Involve neurologist, neurosurgeon. Radiologist and CT scan. ICU and critical outreach team.
Cerebral thrombosis	Headache. Seizures. Neurological deficit as per stroke. Altered conscious level.	Urgent referral. ABC assessment and response. Involve neurologist, neurosurgeon. Radiologist and CT/MRI scan. ICU and critical outreach team.
Cerebral vein thrombosis	Unusually severe headache, which may be associated with neurological focal signs. Confusion. Seizure. Altered conscious level, coma. Most occur postpartum.	Urgent referral. ABC assessment and response. Involve neurologist, radiologist. Require specialist CT/MRI imaging. Treatment with anticoagulation after cerebral bleed excluded. ITU and critical outreach team.
Meningitis	Headache, neck stiffness, vomiting, photophobia, confusion, altered consciousness, seizures, pyrexia, rash.	Urgent referral. ABC assessment and response. Blood cultures and other blood tests. A lumbar puncture may be indicated. Commence antibiotics. ITU, critical outreach team and infection control advice.

continued

Table 9.3 continued

Possible causes of headaches	Features	Actions and investigations
Raised intracranial pressure due to tumour, blocked shunt Idiopathic intracranial hypertension (IIH)	Headache: may be worse in early morning and associated with vomiting. Altered level of consciousness may occur in later stages. Seizures.	Urgent referral as indicated. ABC assessment and response. Involve neurologist, neurosurgeon. Radiologist and CT/MRI scan. ITU and critical outreach team. Medication to reduce intracranial pressure.

with what appears to be a migraine. See the recommended resources at the end of the chapter for discussion of the management of migraine in pregnancy.

In all cases of headache, the midwife should carry out a full set of observations, including assessment for PET, general head-to-toe midwifery assessment and a review of neurological function using AVPU.

Box 9.4 summaries the 'red flag' features of a headache that would indicate a potential serious neurological problem and thus require the midwife to initiate an urgent medical consultation.

Box 9.4 'Red flag' features of a headache that would indicate a potential serious neurological problem and thus require urgent medical referral[13]

- Headache of sudden onset;

- Headache associated with neck stiffness;

- Headache described by the woman as the worst headache she has ever had;

- Headache with any abnormal signs on neurological examination.

Stroke (cerebrovascular accident)

A stroke, also known as a cerebrovascular accident (CVA), is when blood-flow to a part of the brain is stopped, either by a blockage such as a clot (ischaemic stroke) or the rupture of a blood vessel (haemorrhagic stroke). It can result in sudden collapse and rapid deterioration.

The incidence of stroke in pregnancy is about 2–3 times higher when compared with non-pregnant women of childbearing age and a stroke is more likely to occur in the third trimester or in the 6-week postnatal period. It is a devastating event for a pregnant woman and can result in long-term disability or death. In the UK and Ireland between 2009 and 2012, 26 women died of intracerebral haemorrhage.[3] Increasing prevalence of obesity, hypertension and cardiac disease among women of childbearing age may contribute to a higher incidence.[14] Pre-eclampsia (eclampsia in particular) and raised systolic blood pressure contribute to the pathophysiology of stroke related to childbirth in up to 50% of cases.[11,15] See Box 9.5 for risk factors for stroke in pregnancy. A recommendation from the MBRRACE report[3] is that all women experiencing a stroke should be admitted to a hyperacute stroke unit in order to receive urgent specialist care.

Box 9.5 Risk factors for stroke in pregnancy[16,12,17,11]

- The physiological changes that make pregnancy a prothrombotic state: a combination of hypercoagulability, venous stasis and vascular endothelial damage;
- Maternal age greater than 35 years;
- Obesity;
- Hyperlipidaemia;
- History of migraine;
- Smoking;
- Hypertension, pre-eclampsia, eclampsia, HELLP syndrome;
- Diabetes;
- Cardiac conditions;
- Substance abuse (especially cocaine);
- Autoimmune conditions such as systemic lupus erythematosus (SLE) and antiphospholipid syndrome (APS);
- Thrombophilia;
- Sickle cell disease;
- Dehydration;
- Infection and sepsis.

Specific conditions causing stroke in pregnancy

Pre-eclampsia, eclampsia, HELLP

Pre-eclampsia is associated with 25–45% of pregnancy-associated stroke.[16] The pathophysiology of endothelial dysfunction, vasoconstriction and hypertension are factors contributing to a stroke in pregnancy. Both intracerebral haemorrhage and ischaemic events are seen.[16] Increased blood pressure leads to intracranial bleeding. The MBRRACE report 'Saving lives, improving mothers' care 2012–2014'[6] states that there is an urgent need to control severe hypertension and that management should aim to keep women's blood pressure below 150/100.

Because PET is common (2–8% of pregnancies), it is often the most obvious diagnosis in pregnant and postpartum women who present with acute neurological symptoms, and it is common sense to carry out an assessment for PET in these circumstances (see Chapter 6). However, other conditions, such as a stroke or cerebral vein thrombosis, need to be considered to avoid misdiagnosis.

Subarachnoid haemorrhage and rupture of cerebral aneurysm

Subarachnoid haemorrhage (SAH), mostly from rupture of a cerebral aneurysm, accounts for about 3% of strokes related to childbirth.[16] Other causes of SAH include hypertension and eclampsia. The incidence of SAH is greater in pregnancy, although still quite rare (1 in 10,000 pregnancies).[16,17] A sudden and severe 'thunderclap' headache is characteristic. See Table 9.3 for clinical features of subarachnoid haemorrhage.

Cerebral venous thrombosis (CVT)

CVT accounts for about 2% of pregnancy-related stroke and has a high fatality rate. Risks for CVT include hypertension, pre-eclampsia, thrombophilia, infection and dehydration. It is more common in the 3 weeks following delivery.[16,17,11]

Typical presentation includes: headache, vomiting, altered level of consciousness, focal neurological symptoms, photophobia and seizures. Symptoms may develop over several days. Impaired consciousness can range from slight confusion to deep coma.[11]

CVT has the same risk factors as DVT and pulmonary embolism and is linked to the hypercoagulable state of pregnancy (see 'pulmonary embolism' in Chapter 7). In many cases, the woman has an underlying thrombophilia. Possible trauma to the endothelial lining of cerebral vessels during labour may occur. Factors such as dehydration and puerperal infection are also implicated as contributing factors. Treatment includes hydration and anticoagulation.[12]

Seizures

The most common reason for a pregnant or postnatal woman to have a seizure is that she has a pre-existing diagnosis of epilepsy. Seizures can also arise from pregnancy (eclampsia, related to PET) and non-pregnancy-related causes (cerebral damage, metabolic reasons). (See Box 9.6 for causes of seizures in pregnancy in women without known epilepsy.) However, a woman with epilepsy can develop complications such as pre–eclampsia in pregnancy, and, just because she is known to have epilepsy, other causes of seizures should not be ignored. In a woman known to have epilepsy, any

---

Box 9.6 Causes of seizures in pregnancy in women without known epilepsy[12]

- Eclampsia;
- Stroke: cerebral vein thrombosis (CVS), subarachnoid haemorrhage (SAH);
- Previous brain surgery;
- Intracranial mass lesions;
- Antiphospholipid syndrome;
- Thrombotic thrombocytopenia purpura (TTP);
- Drug and alcohol withdrawal;
- Hypoglycaemia (diabetes, hypoadrenalism);
- Hypocalcaemia (magnesium sulphate therapy, hypoparathyroidism);
- Hyponatraemia (hyperemesis);
- Infections (tuberculosis, toxoplasmosis, meningitis, cerebral malaria).

unusual features of the seizures noted by the woman or her family, any increase in frequency or duration of seizures or any other clinical features occurring in conjunction with the seizures would indicate that further investigation and referral are needed.

When a seizure occurs for the first time in pregnancy, a number of investigations are needed (see Box 9.7). The midwife should carry out observations as discussed in section 'Neurological assessment by the midwife'. Box 9.8 summarises the immediate care when a seizure occurs.

Box 9.7 Investigations following a seizure

- Blood pressure, urinalysis and
  other examination for features of PET

Bloods:

- Platelet count, clotting screen and blood film
- Blood glucose
- U&Es
- Renal and liver function tests

Radiology:

- Computerised tomography (CT) or magnetic resonance imaging (MRI) of the brain
- EEG.

Eclampsia

The most common reason for seizure in pregnancy, apart from epilepsy, is eclampsia. Eclampsia is part of the spectrum of disorders featured under the title 'pre-eclampsia' (see Chapter 6). Eclamptic seizures are usually tonic-clonic and last for about 1 minute. They can arise with minimal warning, but the woman may have had a persistent headache, blurred vision, photophobia, epigastric pain and altered mental state beforehand. In up to a third of cases, blood pressure is within normal limits (below 140/90 mmHg) and/or there is no proteinuria.[11] Assessment will include reviewing for signs and symptoms of PET, requesting laboratory tests (PET bloods) and assessing maternal and fetal wellbeing. Treatment with magnesium sulphate has been shown to treat and prevent further seizures.[18] Delivery of the baby is likely to be expedited.

Epilepsy

Epilepsy is the most common neurological disorder to complicate pregnancy. For most women with epilepsy, the disorder predates their pregnancy and is usually managed well with the use of anti-epileptic drugs (AEDs). Seizure type and frequency differs and for most women with epilepsy; pregnancy does not affect the frequency of seizures. However, possible reasons for deterioration in seizure control in pregnancy include:

- Poor compliance with anticonvulsant medication. This is due to fears regarding the development of congenital abnormality linked with AEDs. The recommendation is that women should continue their medication to avoid seizures. Women should access pre-conception assessment so that the lowest dose of suitable medication is prescribed.[12]
- Vomiting in early pregnancy may affect absorption of regular AEDs.
- Physiological changes in pregnancy may affect drug utilisation and clearance.
- Triggers to seizures, such as lack of sleep and stress, may occur more frequently in pregnancy.
- The risk of seizures is highest around the time of birth (approximately 3%).[19] In the MBRRACE[3] review of neurological conditions, 12 women died related to complications of epilepsy; two women drowned, six women died of sudden unexpected death in epilepsy (SUDEP) and four women died following complications of seizures. Pre-conception care, involvement of epilepsy specialist nurses, joint care with specialist services and avoidance of bathing and sleeping alone are some of the recommendations to reduce mortality and morbidity.

Box 9.8 Immediate care of the woman who is having a seizure

- Summon assistance (anaesthetist and obstetrician) urgently.
- Protect from injury during the tonic-clonic phase.
- Maintain airway (clear by suctioning if necessary).
- Provide supplementary oxygenation.
- Place the woman in the left lateral (recovery) position.
- Obtain intravenous access and monitor fluid balance.
- Treat the convulsion: intravenous drugs, usually benzodiazepines (e.g. Lorazepam, Diazepam) and anti-convulsive medication (e.g. Phenytoin), or rectal Diazepam if necessary. If it is possible that seizure is related to PET/eclampsia, magnesium sulphate is recommended.
- Monitor vital signs and beware placental abruption, PPH.
- Achieve stability of maternal condition.
- Assess fetal wellbeing (risk of fetal distress from hypoxia or placental abruption) and evaluate the need for expediting delivery.

Assessment of blood glucose level: hypoglycaemia, ketoacidosis

Both diabetic hypoglycaemia and ketoacidosis can lead to loss of consciousness and coma. Assessing a blood sugar level using a pin prick is a simple and informative test and should be part of the assessment of any woman presenting with confusion or loss of consciousness, regardless of whether she is a known diabetic or not. A high blood sugar can occur as part of the fight-or-flight response in conditions such as sepsis. Normal blood sugar is approximately 4–8 mmol/l.

Hypoglycaemia

Symptoms of hypoglycaemia include feeling hungry, trembling or shakiness, feeling anxious, irritable or moody and sweating. It is known that, in pregnancy, diabetic women may develop hypoglycaemia 'unawareness', and thus a pregnant woman may present in more advanced stages of hypoglycaemia. A mild case of hypoglycaemia, where the woman is able to swallow effectively, can be treated by encouraging her to consume a portion of fast-acting carbohydrate, such as glucose tablets, sweets, sugary fizzy drinks or fruit juice. If she is unable to swallow and/or has a reduced level of consciousness, medical aid should be requested. The midwife, however, should not delay giving an IM injection of glucagon, which will release stored glucose from the liver into the bloodstream, raising the blood sugar level. The woman should be placed into the recovery position, with care taken to maintain a patent airway. Any insulin therapy must be discontinued. When medical help arrives, glucagon or dextrose can be given IV if required. Review glucose levels at frequent intervals to monitor the response to treatment. An insulin administration sliding scale will underpin further management.

Ketoacidosis

Diabetic *ketoacidosis* is a serious complication of diabetes that occurs when there is a lack of insulin. This results in the cells being deprived of the essential glucose needed for cellular energy. Cell starvation triggers an array of metabolic disturbances, which include the production of ketones. Other features of ketoacidosis include: raised blood sugar levels, reduced glycogen stores, excess levels of glycerol and fatty acids and amino acids, increased urine production that results in dehydration and hypovolaemia, low sodium levels and fluctuating potassium levels. The increased oxidation of fatty acids resulting in increasing ketone levels, along with increased lactic acid, result in the life-threatening metabolic acidosis seen in diabetic ketoacidosis.

Ketoacidosis most commonly occurs in conjunction with Type 1 diabetes, but it can also complicate Type 2 diabetes and gestational diabetes mellitus (GDM).[20] Box 9.9 lists the factors that may lead to ketoacidosis in pregnancy. The progression of ketoacidosis can be more rapid in pregnancy, due to the increased insulin resistance

---

Box 9.9 Predisposing/risk factors for ketoacidosis

- Prolonged vomiting and/or starvation;
- Infections;
- Poor control of blood glucose levels (may be caused by poor compliance or insulin pump failure);
- Undiagnosed diabetes;
- Steroid use (prescribed for medical disorders or for fetal lung maturation).

Maternal signs and symptoms are listed in Box 9.10, but it is worth noting that, in one study,[21] 97% included nausea and vomiting in their presenting symptoms.

> **Box 9.10 Signs and symptoms of ketoacidosis**
>
> * Tachypnoea/hyperventilation;
> * Kussmaul respirations (deep, laboured breaths);
> * Smell of acetone (fruity) on breath;
> * Tachycardia;
> * Hypotension;
> * Polyuria/polydipsia/dehydration;
> * Nausea and/or vomiting;
> * Abdominal pain/contractions;
> * Muscle weakness/blurred vision;
> * Changes in behaviour, loss of consciousness and coma.

that occurs in the third trimester. Pregnancy also results in a normal state of respiratory alkalosis, and this is countered by increased renal excretion of bicarbonate. However, this lowered buffering capacity can contribute to ketoacidosis at a lower blood glucose level than is seen in those who are not pregnant.[22]

The metabolic disturbance in the mother will reduce uteroplacental blood flow, overstimulate the fetal pancreas to produce too much insulin and expose the fetus to electrolyte imbalances. Fetal hypoxia and fetal death from arrhythmias may occur. The most effective way to treat the fetus is to treat the mother.[23]

Management requires urgent medical referral and is considered an obstetric emergency. See Table 9.4 for the principles of initial management and ongoing assessment of ketoacidosis

Table 9.4 Initial management and ongoing assessment of ketoacidosis[9]

Where	Call for help – transfer to critical care assessment area as soon as possible.
Multidisciplinary team	Obstetric and midwifery team, anaesthetist, medical team.
Immediate care	Assess ABC – maintain airway, check oxygen saturations and give oxygen as required.
	Lie the woman on left side/left tilt.
	Gain IV access – 2 wide-bore cannulae.
	Check blood sugar levels – capillary testing gives immediate result.
Fluid and drug administration	Treat dehydration – fluid replacement, usually with crystalloids, and normally rapid (e.g.1–2 l in the first 2 hours).
	IV insulin therapy to lower blood glucose levels.
	Correction of abnormal electrolytes.
	Thereafter, may need glucose solution depending on blood results – use insulin sliding scale to guide management.

continued

Table 9.4 continued

Assessment by the medical team	Search for underlying cause – infection, hyperemesis, noncompliance with medication, corticosteroid administration.
Midwifery assessments	Frequent blood sugar measurements to monitor the effectiveness of treatment. Measure BP, pulse, temperature and respirations frequently and record on MEOWS chart. Continuous cardiac monitoring. Urinary catheter: monitor urine output. Test urine for ketones and glucose. Maintain fluid balance chart. Assess fetus wellbeing.
Investigations	Blood tests: renal function tests, FBC, Group and Save, U&Es, random blood sugar and lactate. CRP as part of infection screen. Arterial blood gases.

Further reading

Bothamley, J and Boyle, M. 2009. Medical conditions affecting pregnancy and childbirth. Oxford, UK: Radcliffe Publishing. See Chapter 8, 'Disorders of the nervous system'. Useful information about preconception, antenatal, care in labour and postnatal care for a range of neurological conditions, including epilepsy.

Glasgow Coma Scale website. Available at www.glasgowcomascale.org/. Has a useful video giving detail on how to assess the GCS.

Nelson-Piercy, C. 2015. Handbook of obstetric medicine: management of migraine. Boca Raton, FL: CRC Press. See Chapter 9, 'Neurological problems'. Useful chapter on neurological conditions, including details on the management of epilepsy and migraine.

Teasdale, G. 2014. Forty years on: updating the Glasgow Coma Scale. Nursing Times, 110(42): 12–16. Informative and easy-to-read guide on how to assess the GCS.

References

1. Knight, M, Nour, M, Tuffnell, D, Kenyon, S, Shakespeare, J, Brocklehurst, P and Kurinczuk, JJ (eds) on behalf of MBRRACE-UK. 2016. Saving lives, improving mothers' care: surveillance of maternal deaths in the UK 2012–2014 and lessons learned to inform maternity care from the UK and Ireland Confidential Enquiries into Maternal Deaths and Morbidity 2009–2014. Oxford, UK: National Perinatal Epidemiology Unit, University of Oxford.

2. Knight, M, Tuffnell, D, Kenyon, S, Shakespeare, J, Gray, R and Kurinczuk, JJ (eds) on behalf of MBRRACE-UK. 2015. Saving lives, improving mothers' care: surveillance of maternal deaths in the UK 2011–2013 and lessons learned to inform maternity care from the UK and Ireland confidential enquiries into maternal deaths and morbidity 2009–2013. Oxford, UK: National Perinatal Epidemiology Unit, University of Oxford.

3. Kelso, A and Wills, A on behalf of the MBRRACE-UK neurology chapter writing group. 2014. Learning from neurological complications. In: Knight, M, Kenyon, S, Brocklehurst, P, Neilson, J, Shakespeare, J and Kurinczuk, JJ (eds) on behalf of MBRRACE-UK. Saving lives, improving mothers' care: lessons learned to inform future maternity care from the

UK and Ireland confidential enquiries into maternal deaths and morbidity 2009–2012. Oxford, UK: National Perinatal Epidemiology Unit, University of Oxford, pp. 73–9.

4. Woodrow, P. 2016. *Nursing acutely ill adults.* London: Routledge

5. Scales, K. 2012. The patient with acute neurological problems. In: Peate, I and Dutton, H (eds). *Recognising and responding to medical emergencies.* Harlow, UK: Pearson, pp. 206–39.

6. Harding, K, Redmond, P and Tuffnell, D on behalf of the MBRRACE-UK hypertensive disorders of pregnancy chapter writing group. 2016. Caring for women with hypertensive disorders of pregnancy. In: Knight, M, Nour, M, Tuffnell, D, Kenyon, S, Shakespeare, J, Brocklehurst, P and Kurinczuk, JJ (eds) on behalf of MBRRACE-UK. *Saving lives, improving mothers' care: surveillance of maternal deaths in the UK 2012–2014 and lessons learned to inform maternity care from the UK and Ireland confidential enquiries into maternal deaths and morbidity 2009–2014.* Oxford, UK: National Perinatal Epidemiology Unit, University of Oxford, pp. 69–75.

7. Woodrow, P. 2009. Neurological assessment. In: Moore, T and Woodrow, P (eds). *High dependency nursing care: observation, intervention and support for Level 2 patients.* London: Routledge, pp. 77–84.

8. Teasdale, G, Maas, A Leckey, F, Manley, G, Stocchetti, N and Murray, G. 2014. The Glasgow Coma Scale at 40 years: standing the test of time. *The Lancet Neurology, 13*(8): 844–54.

9. Paterson-Brown, S and Howell, C (eds). 2014. *The Moet Course Manual: managing obstetric emergencies and trauma.* Cambridge, UK: Cambridge University Press.

10. Resuscitation Council (UK). 2015. Adult basic life support and automated external defibrillation. Available at www.resus.org.uk/resuscitation-guidelines/adult-basic-life-support-and-automated-external-defibrillation/. Accessed 27 September 2017.

11. Edlow, JA, Caplan, LR, O'Brien, K and Tibbles, CD. 2013. Diagnosis of acute neurological emergencies in pregnant and postpartum women. *The Lancet Neurology, 12*(2): 175–85.

12. Nelson-Piercy, C. 2015. *Handbook of obstetric medicine.* Boca Raton, FL: CRC Press.

13. Oates, M, Harper, A, Shakespeare, J and Nelson-Piercy, C. 2011. Back to basics. In: Centre for Maternal and Child Enquiries (CMACE) (eds). Saving mothers' lives: reviewing maternal deaths to make motherhood safer: 2006–2008. The eighth report of the confidential enquiries into maternal deaths in the United Kingdom. *British Journal of Obstetrics and Gynaecology, 118*(1): s1–203.

14. Moatti, Z, Gupta, M, Yadava, R and Thamban, S. 2014. A review of stroke and pregnancy: incidence, management and prevention. *European Journal of Obstetrics and Gynecology: Reproductive Biology, 181*: 20–7. doi: 10.1016/j.ejogrb.2014.07.024.

15. Caplan, LR and Haussen, DC. 2016. Stroke in pregnancy. In: Klein, A, O'Neal, A, Scifres, C, Waters, JF and Waters, JH (eds). *Neurological illness in pregnancy and practice.* Cichester, UK: John Wiley & Sons, pp. 92–109.

16. Narayan, H. 2015. *Compendium for antenatal care of high risk pregnancies.* Oxford, UK: Oxford University Press.

17. Carhuapoma, JR, Tomlinson, MW and Levine, SR. 2011. Neurological complications. In: James, D (ed.). *High risk pregnancy: management options.* St Louis, MO: Elsevier.

18. The Magpie Trial Collaborative Group. 2002. Do women with pre-eclampsia, and their babies, benefit from magnesium sulphate? The Magpie Trial: a randomised placebo-controlled trial. *Lancet, 359*(9321):1877–90.

19. Battino, D, Tomson, T, Bonizzoni, E, Craig, J, Lindhout, D, Sabers, A, Perucca E and Vajda, F on behalf of the EURAP study group. 2013. Seizure control and treatment changes in pregnancy: observations from the EURAP epilepsy pregnancy registry. *Epilepsia, 54*(9): 1621–7.

20. Landon, M and Gabbe, S. 2011. Gestational diabetes mellitus. *Obstetrics and Gynecology,* *118*(6): 1379–93.

21. Bryant, S, Herrera, C, Nelson, D and Cunningham, F. 2017. Diabetic ketoacidosis complicating pregnancy. *Journal of Neonatal–Perinatal Medicine, 10*(1): 17–23

22. Guo, R, Yang, L, Li, L and Shao, X. 2008. Diabetic ketoacidosis in pregnancy tends to occur at lower blood glucose levels: case-control study and a case report of euglycemic diabetic ketoacidosis in pregnancy. *Journal of Obstetrics and Gynaecology Research, 34*(3): 324–30.

23. Sibai, B and Viteri, O. 2014. Diabetic ketosacidosis in pregnancy. *American College of Obstetricians and Gynecologists, 123*(1): 167–78.

Glossary

Acidosis: an extremely acidic condition caused by overproduction of acid in the blood or an excessive loss of bicarbonate from the blood (metabolic acidosis), or by a build-up of carbon dioxide in the blood from poor lung function or depressed breathing (respiratory acidosis).

Anoxia: lack of oxygen overall.

Anuria: failure of the kidneys to produce urine.

AVPU assessment: basic neurological assessment (alert/responds to verbal stimuli/responds to painful stimuli/unresponsive)

Bradycardia: in an adult, a heart rate < 60 bpm. Fetal bradycardia is < 110 bpm.

Bradypnoea: in an adult, respirations < 12. In a newborn, respirations < 40.

Capillary refill test: test of the time taken for colour to return to an external capillary after occlusion, normally done on fingertips.

Clonus: a large or repetitive muscular reaction from reflex or stretching.

Coagulopathy: when the blood's ability to coagulate (form clots) is impaired.

Complement system: part of the immune system that enhances the ability of antibodies and phagocytic cells to clear microbes/damaged cells, promotes inflammation and attacks pathogens.

Crepitation: a crackling or rattling sound from lungs/breathing.

Cyanosis: blue discoloration due to hypoxaemia.

Dyspnoea: difficulty in breathing.

Encephalopathy: a disorder or disease of the brain.

Fulminate: a very rapid (and usually severe) progression of a disease.

Haemoptysis: coughing up blood.

Hyperkalaemia: high potassium.

Hypoxaemia: low oxygen in the blood.

Hypoxia: inadequate oxygen at cellular level.

Kinin system: hormonal system that plays a role in inflammation, blood pressure control, coagulation and pain.

Oliguria: reduced urine output.

Orthopnoea: shortness of breath when lying flat.

Papilloedema: congestion of optic disc.

Paroxysmal nocturnal dyspnoea: being woken when asleep by a feeling of SOB.

Platypnoea: shortness of breath when sitting upright.

Pleuritic chest pain: a sharp chest pain occurring with deep breaths, which may become worse with coughs, sneezes or movement.

Polycythaemia: a high red blood cell count.

Polydipsia: excessive thirst.

Polyuria: excessive urination.

Pulse pressure: the difference between the systolic and diastolic pressure readings.

Stridor: high-pitched, wheezing sound caused by disrupted airflow during respiration.

Supine hypotension syndrome: when the gravid uterus impedes the inferior vena cava and venous return.

Syncope: fainting

Tachycardia: in an adult, a heart rate > 100 bpm. Fetal tachycardia is > 160 bpm.

Tachypnoea: in an adult, a respiratory rate > 20 per minute, in a newborn > 60 per minute.

Thrombocytopenia: low blood platelet count.

Thrombophilia: a condition where the blood has an increased tendency to form clots.

Urticarial: rash of round, red wheals on the skin that itch intensely, sometimes with dangerous swelling. Caused by an allergic reaction, typically to specific foods.

Index

Note: *italics* indicate figures; **bold** indicates tables and boxes.

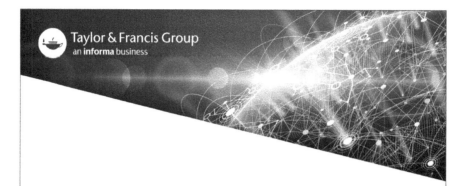

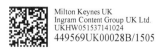
Milton Keynes UK
Ingram Content Group UK Ltd.
UKHW051537141024
449569UK00028B/1505